THE
NATURAL
HEALTH
SERVICE

How Nature Can
Mend Your Mind

ISABEL
HARDMAN

Atlantic Books
London

First published in hardback and trade paperback in Great Britain in 2020 by Atlantic Books, an imprint of Atlantic Books Ltd.

This edition published in 2021.

10 9 8 7 6 5 4 3 2 1

A CIP catalogue record for this book is available from the British Library.

Paperback ISBN: 978 1 78649 592 1
E-book ISBN: 978 1 78649 593 8

Printed and bound by CPI Group (UK) Ltd, Croydon CR0 4YY

Atlantic Books
An imprint of Atlantic Books Ltd
Ormond House
26–27 Boswell Street
London
WC1N 3JZ

www.atlantic-books.co.uk

'A vigorous case for nature as the great healer we have overlooked.'
Financial Times

'Robustly argued... Elation comes in many forms: an unexpected orchid in a Glasgow car park, a shy kingfisher by the Thames, and Penny Black, a headstrong pony in Wimbledon.'
Observer

'Hardman is a precise, lucid writer, never afraid to offer well-argued opinion but always careful to delineate it from factual reporting... *The Natural Health Service* is rich in interesting and unusual details.'
The Critic

'A compelling and passionately argued case that healthy bodies and minds need nature.'
The Lancet

'A really uplifting book. Amid the vivid depictions of depression and PTSD there is a joy in these pages as Isabel explains what the natural world has given to her, and can give to all of us.'
Alastair Campbell

'Absorbing and life-affirming... Isabel's journey of discovery through her own mental illness contains lessons for us all. Simply a must-read.'
Rachel Cullen

'Extraordinary. I wish everyone with a mental illness, and all those supporting them, would read this book. I believe it could help to revolutionise the way we think about, and even treat, mental health issues.'
Jonny Benjamin MBE

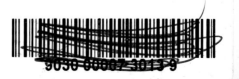

Isabel Hardman is a journalist, author and broadcaster. She is Assistant Editor of the *Spectator* and presents *Week in Westminster* on BBC Radio 4. In 2015 she was named Journalist of the Year at the Political Studies Association's annual awards. She is the author of the bestseller *Why We Get the Wrong Politicians* which won at the 2018 Parliamentary Book Awards and was shortlisted for Waterstones Book of the Year. She is a prominent campaigner on mental health and lives in London.

Contents

Preface to the Paperback Edition

No one could have predicted the circumstances in which this book was first published. It was supposed to appear on bookshop shelves just as the weather was improving and spring leaves opening. It would be easy for people to put into practice the lessons about getting outdoors regularly to help their mental health.

But instead, the bookshops were closed and people were being told by the government and the police to stay at home to stop the spread of coronavirus. And yet, so many of our experiences in 2020 underlined the central arguments of this book.

While we couldn't see our family or friends, or go into work, or visit 'non-essential' shops, one of the few things most people were still allowed to do, even at the height of lockdown, was get out of the house and do some socially-distanced exercise. The medical experts were adamant that there was an important link between outdoor exercise and wellbeing, both physical and mental. The behavioural psychologists were adamant that the once-daily outdoor exercise would help people stick to other restrictions better. The politicians agreed.

Lockdown was such a strange time that few were able to take a step back and note quite how extraordinary this was. Outdoor exercise had gone from a hobby or something to fill your free time to being an important part of the effort to fight COVID-19. It was no longer a niche luxury, but an essential. Of course, the professionals and patients who I had interviewed for *The Natural Health Service* already had that attitude, but it was not prevalent in the general population until 2020.

Coronavirus has forced society to change at a speed it isn't normally capable of. Even old-fashioned companies have realised that home working doesn't necessarily mean a plunge in productivity. In the UK, normally thrifty Conservative politicians have discovered a love of spending vast amounts of money. And what might have been a dawning realisation about the value of nature for all of our good health became an epiphany for so many.

In the early days of lockdown, I encouraged people on social media to try connecting with nature in a different way each day, even if they were forced to shield at home. I was struck by how many almost had to retune themselves to a new frequency in order to do so. One day, I suggested looking out of the window and taking a photo of the nearest tree. A number of people responded with photos of trees in their streets that they had never even noticed before, confessing that they had thought it was a shame they had no greenery outside their window, before realising that they had just failed to notice it. Others reported that for the first time in their lives, they were leaving the house every day for a walk. They came to rely on this so much for sanity that they were determined to continue the habit long after COVID-19 was under control.

It wasn't an easy transition, though. In the UK, local authorities panicked and closed parks, and politicians seemed genuinely surprised by the disparity in access to green space between the fortunate and those on low incomes. It was much easier to be locked down with a garden, for instance, but rather harder in a tower block. I watched as this book became an important part of the push for better access to green spaces, and against suggestions, from some quarters, that restrictions be tightened to the extent that people wouldn't be able to go more than 100 metres from their homes, as had been the case in some other European countries.

We now know that life isn't going to go back to the old normal anytime soon. There are many bad things about this, but one good thing is that we have an opportunity to change the way we live and the importance we place on the great outdoors and exercising within it. We shouldn't go back to seeing it as an optional extra in the treatment of mental health problems, or, indeed, as something to pay lip service to when planning towns, homes and workplaces.

The problem is that mental health services are now even more stretched than they were when I started writing *The Natural Health Service*. People are having to wait longer, for what is often a worse quality of treatment, as a result of the backlog and raised demand caused by the pandemic. Politicians continue to speak worthy words about mental health, but they are still failing to fund it adequately.

The lifting of restrictions also highlighted how poor outdoor literacy is for many people. Britain's nature reserves and beauty spots reported an influx of illegal campers who left disgraceful amounts of litter in their wake. It wasn't clear whether the offenders were used to leaving their junk all over the place in beautiful locations overseas, whether they were more used to camping at festivals, which often end with a sea of abandoned tents, or whether they genuinely had no idea that beauty spots don't stay lovely for very long if you start trashing them. Some people have a selfish attitude towards the natural world: it exists purely for them as individuals so they treat it with no more respect than a cheap item of fast fashion. We have spent much of the past few months talking about the need to protect the NHS. COVID-19 has shown how much we need to protect the Natural Health Service too, so that it is still available for those whose minds need mending, as well as ourselves.

For my own part, a few days after this book was first published, I gave birth to a son. My life has changed a great deal, but one thing remains the same: I need to be outdoors to stay healthy. The challenges are different, of course: I rarely have both hands free at once and I have to plan with even greater determination so that I make it to the riverbank for a swim, or so that I am able to go for a run. I know I can cope better with the days when I have had little sleep and my baby is not in good humour if I have gone outside for a walk, or if I have had a dip. And despite all the demands of motherhood with a mental illness, I am even more confident now that the great outdoors is something that can be fitted into every kind of life, whether gloriously free of responsibilities, or wonderfully busy tending to a child. It will sustain me for the rest of my life; and in time I hope my son will grow up to say the same. I hope that by the time he is an adult, the Natural Health Service is such common parlance that, as with our established NHS, we will all wonder how we got along without it.

Isabel Hardman, September 2020

Madness and Orchidelirium

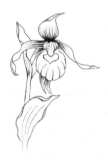

It was only when I was lost for words that I realised how ill I was. I wasn't just going through a bad few months, in need of another week off here and a half day there. I was really, really sick, needing emergency treatment, sedation and years of recovery. Words were how I made a living: thousands of them every day on what British politicians were up to now. I was garrulous: long car journeys across the country could be taken up with all the words I had to offer, on any subject, pausing only when friends managed to interject. Fellow journalists had special words to describe my work ethic, such as 'Stakhanovite'. Every day I was bursting with more words. But one evening in September 2016, the words just stopped coming. I found myself staring at a blank computer screen with half a sentence of what was supposed to be another 500 words or so on British politics. I couldn't string the rest of it together.

Maybe it was that my head was so noisy that the words couldn't find their way out. I had been diagnosed with anxiety and depression three months before and, despite being prescribed what newspapers would call 'a cocktail of drugs', I wasn't getting any better. I had been finding it increasingly hard to focus on just one thing: I couldn't follow what people were saying at work or even during the sort of trashy TV programmes we all watch at the end of a long day because they're so easy to understand. Instead, my mind was constantly on a washing machine spin cycle of bad thoughts: paranoia about what the people around me were going to do; endless rumination over things that had happened in my past that I had no way of changing; and, increasingly, a desire to hurt myself or turn myself off entirely.

Looking back, it isn't at all surprising that I ended up so ill. I'd experienced a serious trauma in my past. The temptation now is just to write more about that, but I'm not sure I'll ever be well enough to publicly relive what happened, and this isn't intended to be one of those miserable books. But it was bad enough to make the jaws of healthcare professionals sag a little in shock whenever I told them. It made one of my burliest friends cry when I told him. I still notice the fists of family members clench with horror whenever the subject comes up.

My approach to recovering from this trauma at the time was totally stupid yet also alarmingly common. I decided that the best way to deal with what had happened was just to try to get on with things, despite my employer offering me compassionate leave. After one of the worst nights of my life, I actually cycled to work early so I could cover the Budget, and pretended to my colleagues that absolutely nothing had happened. I then tried to soldier through covering the EU referendum, the brutal murder of an MP, endless party leadership contests (the UK Independence Party (UKIP) became completely addicted to the things), and the seemingly eternal madness unleashed upon British politics ever since. My healthy colleagues struggled to sleep or see their children. I ended up having a mental breakdown.

My mind, something that up to this point had got me into a series of fulfilling and demanding jobs in journalism, felt as though it was wandering off in all sorts of directions, ignoring my pleas for it to return to whatever I was trying to concentrate on. All of us have strange, intrusive thoughts that fly into our heads from time to time. But a well person can send them on their way with a cerebral shrug. Instead, my obsessive, frightening thoughts settled like a parliament of rooks, noisily distracting me from anything and everything.

I started taking antidepressants on my doctor's advice, and waited for them to work. Nothing seemed to be helping. Even a holiday in Nice didn't improve things: I had just started seeing my partner John and we decided to get away for a weekend for a rest. Instead, we found ourselves surrounded by screaming crowds as people ran for their lives from the Bastille Day attack on the Promenade des Anglais. When we returned to the site two days later, we found the bulk of floral tributes marking the spots where people had fallen. They were lying in the very place where we had, just five or ten minutes earlier, been watching fireworks and enjoying the happy chatter of those around us. Near misses make you appreciate what you could have so easily and quickly lost. But they also stop you relaxing.

I was still trying to work on the day of my breakdown.

I was at the Conservative Party conference in Birmingham, which is one of the biggest events for a journalist like me. At the previous week's Labour conference in Liverpool, panic attacks were coming so thick and fast that I could barely leave my bedroom. I was trying to give my colleagues the impression that I was as reliable as ever, but, looking back, it must have been a terribly unconvincing performance.

One evening as I tried to write the political briefing that I'd sent every day for the past four years of working at the *Spectator*, I realised that my mind had just stopped working. I couldn't string a sentence together, even though this email, read by everyone from the Prime Minister down, usually only took me about thirty minutes to put together. After an hour, I had managed just a few words and was beginning to understand the meaning of 'gibbering wreck'. I was supposed to be speaking at a dinner after this, then appearing on TV, but all I could do was call John and mutter terrified phrases down the phone.

I ended up being sedated that night, and shuffled my way home the next morning to start two months of sick leave. Over the coming years I swung between sick leave and trying to settle back down at my desk to get some work done. Slowly, the words came back, timidly at first, and then roosting neatly in a line so that I could write sentences again. In time, I wrote a book. And then a second one (this one, in fact). I tend not to think too much about whether

I'm 'better' yet, not least because I don't really know what that word means. Everyone – from me to my employer to my partner and my family – has had to accept that I'm not going to go back to who I once was. But mostly I can work, write books, cover politics for British publications and broadcasters, and, most gloriously, string a sentence together.

I wouldn't have got to this stage of 'better' without the NHS – just not the one you imagine I'm talking about. The English National Health Service did do a great deal to help me recover from the most acute phases of what turned out to be post-traumatic stress disorder (PTSD). It prescribed me medication (though it took months to find the right pill), kept an eye on how I was managing and tried its best to direct me to therapy. I wouldn't be here without the GP who kept booking double appointments so she could really find out what I was up to and whether the latest prescription was working or making things worse, or indeed without the Accident and Emergency doctors who kept me safe and helped me get more support in the community. But there was another health service which intervened in my recovery with even more dramatic results: the Natural Health Service – a great outdoors which made me want to keep living, and made living much more bearable.

I came across this almost by accident. One of the things no one tells you about being mentally ill is how dreadfully boring it is. You can't do the normal things that drive your life along: you're not working and you can't imagine seeing friends and trying to keep up with their conversation, like the child at the back of a school cross-country race. It's even worse if you're an inpatient in a hospital as you don't always have Internet access or a TV to watch. And so you end up trying to find things to keep you busy. About a year after first falling ill, I was back on long-term sick leave once again, floating miserably around our home in Barrow-in-Furness, Cumbria. John was the local MP and fighting an election we hadn't expected would be called. He assumed he would lose, but was out on doorsteps or at campaign events and hustings all day long. I wasn't well enough to cover this snap election – all my words had flown off again – and so I had to find something to do with the very long, lonely days.

I'd been reading about a Victorian craze called 'Orchidelirium': literally orchid madness. Many people are still a little loopy about orchids: they form the largest and most bizarre plant families on earth, ranging from those showy moth orchids that so many of us end up killing on our windowsills to tiny little green flowers that prefer to hang out in bogs.

But while they might be popular today, previous generations were utterly bonkers about these plants, to the extent that they drove some of them to extinction. The most famous British victim of Orchidelirium was the lady's-slipper orchid. This doesn't look like it should belong in Europe, let alone the rugged Yorkshire Dales, where the last surviving wild specimen still grows under twenty-four-hour surveillance to protect it from the clutches of collectors. Its parts barely look as though they belong together: a fat, acid-yellow, slipper-like lip (more of a clog) surrounded by regal claret-coloured petals and corkscrew-twisting sepals. It even has a beautifully exotic perfume, and yet it has long been native to the British Isles. Plant collectors loved the lady's-slipper orchid to death: they dug it up until it had disappeared totally from the wild. In 1917, it was declared extinct.

But then in 1930, one turned up in the Yorkshire Dales, and since then the plant world has gone a little mad once again trying to protect it. There's a warden, a secret committee, trip wires and high fences all to prevent one plant from slipping away from existence. In the meantime, scientists worked out a way of propagating the lady's-slipper and reintroduced it at other wild sites. One of them, I discovered, was just down the road from me. Which was how I ended up trying out Orchidelirium.

I needed to find something that had nothing to do with work to distract myself from the torture chamber in my mind, and so I decided to explore the countryside that surrounded our home in Barrow. Cumbria is one of the best counties in England for wild orchids, competing only with Kent for species. And just over the border in Lancashire was one of the only publicly accessible sites for lady's-slipper orchids. I had nothing else to do: I might as well go orchid-hunting.

The first time I saw those orchids at the Gait Barrows National Nature Reserve in Silverdale, I forgot how bad I was feeling for about twenty minutes; I was so excited to have seen something so strange, with such an extraordinary story of survival and madness behind it. I wanted to find more orchids and learn about the strange wild flowers growing all around me. Plants are the basis of all life on earth and are often so simple that we overlook them. Yet these simple things had made me realise, for the first time in weeks, that there was still something to be appreciated in life. And my desire to see more of it gave me a retort to the suicidal thoughts that kept trying to wrap themselves around me.

I'd already learned that being active outdoors was important. I knew very well that missing a dose of my antidepressant sertraline would have an effect, but so would failing to get outside. I was lucky to have a GP who insisted on probing me about what else I was getting up to. In the days after my breakdown in 2016, she asked me to tell her what I really enjoyed doing in my spare time. I'd grown up a country girl who rode horses in every spare minute, and had started to enjoy running in my late twenties. The doctor listened, and told me that I should arrange riding lessons and running sessions that it would be hard to duck out of. She was worried that, without a booking, I'd just stay indoors, festering mentally.

Even in my foggy sick state back in 2016, I was angered by how much money was seemingly required to get better. It was fine for me, as I could just about afford it, but who has savings these days? After a few months of trying to recover and missing work, I didn't, either. The final chapter of this book will look at ways of preventing the great outdoors from ever being something that only the well-off can use to manage their mental health problems. Likewise, every single chapter will focus on low-cost or free activities as mental illness does not respect class or the size of your savings account. But, once again, it is an example of how poorly we treat mental illness. When we do hit on something that might work, we don't then realise that this activity might be prohibitively expensive to someone whose mental illness means they cannot work, for instance.

My GP was right, though, that I needed help getting out of the door. Without a cheery woman called Vanda appearing at my front door twice a week and talking to me as I puffed my drugged-up way through the streets of south-west London, and without Rhea, a lovely sensible pony in Wimbledon who even sorted me out on a day when I'd been considering how I might kill myself, I wouldn't have had a chance to return to work as a political journalist so I could write about the injustices I had seen first-hand in our health system. The doctor hadn't just handed out prescriptions of pills in my case: she'd also prescribed some time in the great outdoors.

By the following year, I was relying on the Natural Health Service so much that I began to wonder whether there might be something in it for other people, too.

CHAPTER ONE

Why We Need Nature

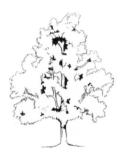

Across the world, there is a growing movement towards using the outdoors in the treatment of a range of mental illnesses, whether it be government-backed forest-bathing centres in Japan, horses conducting therapy sessions in Australia or doctors handing out 'outdoor prescriptions' in Britain. This book is going to explore not just the evidence for obsessing about orchids, or cold-water swimming, or walking in a forest, but also what our policymakers can do to make the Natural Health Service as obvious an intervention in mental healthcare as the pills and the therapy. The great outdoors could be our greatest untapped lifeline.

We will meet many people with mental health problems, and many of the professionals who treat them. They have generously spoken to me, some on the condition of anonymity, in order to help others with their illnesses. Hopefully it will be clear from the case studies that there is no one cause of mental ill health, and that sometimes it's not particularly clear whether there was one discrete 'cause' at all. I have outlined a little of the background to my illness, but like many of the others featured in this book, I don't want to tell the full story, nor do I think it would help the reader particularly to know it. Similarly, I have avoided going into too much detail on my symptoms, partly because there are some things I would rather not relive. This has been the case for many of those I spoke to, and while this may mean there are still questions about what feels like an incomplete example, this is just how it has to be when sharing mental health problems with such a wide audience. There is a difficult boundary between showing honesty to help others (and, often, ourselves) and the need for privacy to protect ourselves too. Each person sets that boundary in a slightly different place, but the purpose of this book is not to educate you in my individual misery, but to show how powerful the great outdoors can be.

Of course, the idea that nature and outdoor exercise can be good for your soul is hardly new. Plato was apparently rather keen on the way exercise helped the mind, and a quote attributed to the philosopher says: 'In order for man to succeed in life, God provided him with two means, education and physical activity. Not separately, one for the soul and the other for the body, but for the two together. With these means, man can attain perfection.'[1] Not a snappy enough quote to find its way on to Instagram, but you get the point.

More recently, the catchily titled *British Manly Exercises*, written by Donald Walker and published in 1834, agreed.[2] This manual insisted that exercise could not only improve physical health, but also make people happier. Walker wrote that outdoor exercise was good for 'the mental faculties'.

Walker wasn't alone in this belief when he was writing. In the long line of paintings hanging in the National Portrait Gallery in London, one stands out. It's not just that the subject is a woman, which is rare enough in itself – it's the fierce, far-sighted look in her eyes, the proud bearing of someone who has lived a life far more noble than some of those she sits alongside. Yet given the impact her work and ideas had on modern Britain, Octavia Hill is astonishingly little-known. She was a pioneer of social housing, getting deeply involved in her tenants' lives as she tried to reform them. She was one of the founders of modern social work and also believed passionately in the great outdoors.

Hill's love of open spaces stemmed from her time spent in places that were the very opposite: dark, dingy, dangerous slum housing which she felt made it even more difficult for the people she cared for to have decent, happy lives. In a newspaper article titled 'Space For The People', she wrote rather forcefully about the difference outdoor space could make to the people she worked with:

> Sometimes on such a hot summer evening in such a court when I am trying to calm excited women shouting their execrable language at one another, I have looked up suddenly and seen one of those bright gleams of light the summer sun sends out just before he sets, catching

the top of a red chimney-pot, and beautiful there, though too directly above their heads for the crowd below to notice it much. But to me it brings sad thought of the fair and quiet places far away, where it is falling softly on tree, and hill, and cloud, and I feel as if that quiet, that beauty, that space, would be more powerful to calm the wild excess about me than all my frantic striving with it.[3]

She called for 'places to sit in, places to play in, places to stroll in, and places to spend a day in', and said that even costly land for housing in London had greater value as outdoor space: 'To my mind they are even now worth very much; but they will be more and more valuable every year – valuable in the deepest sense of the word; health-giving, joy-inspiring, peace-bringing.'

Hill wasn't a particularly fluffy character. You wouldn't find her tweeting life-affirming memes involving pictures of sunsets, even though she clearly believed that those sunsets could do a great deal of good in life. She was a true force of nature and, in being so, was a force for nature too. Some of the greatest green spaces in London are still open and safe today thanks to her campaigning. Hampstead Heath and Parliament Hill Fields, both of which feature later in this book as places where many men and women still restore their minds, were saved from development by her and others. So were areas around London which Hill called the 'Green Belt', a term we still use and debate regularly today. A campaign with John Ruskin to save the fells above Buttermere in Cumbria from development led to the pair hatching a plan for a trust that would conserve beautiful open spaces and historic buildings. Hill wanted to call it the 'Commons and Gardens Trust', but her legal adviser

Sir Robert Hunter put forward the name 'National Trust'. And that's what it became.

More recently, though, proper research has come along to back up our centuries-old hunches about the great outdoors. Researchers in the 1970s and 1980s carried out a small study involving forty-six patients recovering from gall bladder surgery in a Pennsylvania hospital.[4] Half of those patients had rooms whose windows faced a 'natural scene', while the other half could only see a brick wall. The study found that those who could see the natural landscape took fewer powerful painkillers, stayed in hospital for a shorter amount of time after the operation and did better when being assessed by the nurses. Similarly, prisoners whose cells had a natural view were less stressed and were less likely to need medical attention.[5]

But it's not just physical illness that benefits from nature. Over the past few decades, researchers have found that contact with nature, whether through windows or as someone's immediate surroundings, can:

- reduce anxiety and stress[6]
- improve mood[7]
- raise self-esteem
- improve psychological well-being[8]

Some of the work in recent years has been exciting, and hopeful: it suggests that we can use the great outdoors to help our minds in a way that can, at times, be even more powerful than the pills we take.

Why the outdoors in particular? There are many indoor activities that people with mental illnesses swear by: art therapy, music, reading and dancing to name a few. But some researchers believe that being outdoors supercharges therapeutic activities to the extent that we heal better and notice the pain a little less as we go. Therapists who we will meet throughout this book agree with that point about the value of the outside in getting someone to open their mouth for the first time and explain what's going on inside. Some projects even make the natural world a central part of their treatment: when we visit Operation Centaur in Chapter Seven, we will see how horses help people who find it very hard to talk about the problems causing their addictions. Horses can't talk, and yet without one rambling around in front of the patient, the therapist can't get started.

There are plenty of theories about why nature has a particular power over the mind. Many of them run along the lines that we as humans are part of nature and have evolved alongside it, and therefore our natural state is *in* nature. American biologist Edward O. Wilson argues that the profound effect of the great outdoors on humans is as a result of our innate connection to the natural world. This hypothesis argues that humans have an 'innate tendency to focus on life and lifelike processes' because they have evolved alongside or even as part of nature. Wilson points to the unconscious ways people gravitate towards nature by visiting zoos, spending more money on homes above water and surrounded by parkland, and by 'dreaming of snakes for reasons they cannot explain'.[9] So we are most ourselves in nature because nature has been an essential part of human existence. There's even a term for it – 'biophilia' – coined by social psychologist Erich Fromm, which Wilson then took up to explain why it is that we respond to nature in a certain way. There are other names for it, too: if you want to sound like the sort of trendy person who watches Scandi films and furnishes their home according to hygge principles, then try the Nordic 'friluftsliv', which refers to the healing power of nature and humans' need to be in the great outdoors. Biophilia helps us understand why we feel calmer when we look through the window at the trees outside, and even why that phrase 'get back to nature' is so compelling, even for city dwellers. It sounds like a posh word for what is common sense, but if we do think that humans have an innate connection to nature because we have evolved alongside and as part of it, we're not doing a very good job of living out that conviction. We do not design our homes or towns with this deep emotional need in mind, and we certainly don't structure our working lives around it. Most workplaces that aren't dicing with employment law accept that workers need to go to the toilet and eat lunch. But there are few that see a connection to nature as being even vaguely important to their staff, save perhaps the odd garden centre or slightly annoying social media giant.

But understanding that nature isn't merely incidental to our lives helps explain why there is so much power behind so many of the interventions in this book. If the biophilia hypothesis is correct, then why should it be a surprise that so many people find doing therapy outdoors much less daunting than between the four walls of a counselling room? It also has profound implications for the way we live that go far beyond the treatment of clinical problems and into what we consider to be good mental hygiene for every person.

This innate connection to the natural world could even mean that our minds heal when in the outdoors. Environmental psychologists Stephen and Rachel Kaplan have developed a theory called 'Attention

Restoration Theory' (ART).[10] ART states that time spent in nature can renew our attention spans when they are flagging after a hard day's work – or an extended period staring at a screen. Their theory includes four stages of attention restoration in nature, which starts with our minds clearing of the things we've been focusing on and worrying about. Then the mental fatigue that we are suffering from as a result of the hard focus on work or a phone begins to lift. After that, we experience soft fascination, which involves paying attention without any real effort to the things around us, such as the sound of the bird, the view in front of us, water moving through a stream. Finally, we find ourselves relaxing to the point that our attention is restored and we are then able to think about our lives in a more constructive manner. Research suggests that we find it easier to resolve minor life problems when spending time in natural settings.[11]

Similarly, it shouldn't really come as a surprise that running helps your mind and your body, unless you've ended up assuming that the two are completely separate and can never influence one another. If you have, you're in good company. It is only recently that society, and even the medical establishment, has started to acknowledge that our physical health and our mental health aren't as separate as we assumed. Some medics now believe that the Cartesian divide between the two has limited our ability to understand the causes of illnesses such as depression, believing that they must be 'all in the mind', rather than perhaps related to the immune system or other physical processes. Breaking down that divide could have profound consequences for medical research, but on a more basic level, it also now means that we commonly accept that running, for instance, isn't just good for your physical fitness but also your mental state. So much of this book is about doing things, rather than thinking things. One benefits the other.

Social Prescribing

My GP wasn't the only doctor telling their depressed patients that they needed to get out more. Social prescribing is becoming more and more popular in primary care as doctors try to make medicine about the lives that their patients lead and not just about the pills they pop. It involves a doctor referring someone on to a local activity that they feel will benefit their health, and not just their mental health. GPs write social prescriptions for people who suffer from rheumatoid arthritis, for instance, which disproves the observation that being prescribed a good run just shows there isn't that much wrong with you after all.

In 2018, NHS Shetland shot to attention when it ordered its GPs to give 'nature prescriptions' to several patients with debilitating physical and mental health problems. Doctors handed out lists of bird walks and outdoor activities to work alongside their prescriptions for pills. January's prescriptions included: 'really look at a lichen', 'walk the core path at Lunga Water – look out for mountain hares' and 'step outside – be still for three minutes and listen'. In August, patients were told to learn about seaweeds, 'turn o'er a rock and see what you see' and 'try "charming" a worm from the ground without digging or adding liquids… rhythm is the answer'.

The Shetland doctors reckoned they were the first to be handing out such formal nature-based prescriptions, but a less specific form of social prescribing has been going on for a lot longer. Helen Stokes-Lampard was Chair of the Royal College of General Practitioners, between 2016 and 2019, and made social prescribing one of her priorities. She argues that 'social prescribing is just a fancy way of saying what GPs have been doing all the time' in that doctors often end up helping people with problems that can't always be treated with medicine itself: 'It is not my job as a GP to be someone's friend, their counsellor and so on. It is my job to identify what those patients need, and have places to refer people on to.'

The most famous social prescribing practice is the Bromley by Bow Centre in south-east London. The centre takes referrals from GPs of people who have problems that medicine can't tackle, and helps those patients with money, housing or employment problems, as well as prescribing them walking, running, drama, yoga and so on. The doctors who use the service are stridently positive about it, with 95 per cent saying that social prescribing brought well-being to their patients, and 98 per cent feeling it brought well-being to them in their profession, too, presumably because the underlying problems that kept sending their patients back into their surgery were actually being addressed.[12]

The Royal College of Psychiatrists believes that social prescribing can potentially help anyone with any kind of mental illness, including those with severe and enduring conditions which mean they spend a lot of time as inpatients. Dr Katherine Kennet is a sustainability scholar for the College and is insistent that as government ministers become more interested in social prescribing, they must not start to see it as something that can replace more costly talking therapies and medication. She says:

Social prescribing is not an alternative. If you have a severe and enduring illness, there is a lot of evidence that medication and therapy really have a role. And social prescribing isn't about a doctor saying 'take more walks'. It's sending that patient to their link worker, who then sits down for an hour or so with them and works out their interests and what might work for them from the available local resources/ groups. The link worker might go to the project with the patient if their illness means it's hard for them to feel as though they can turn up for the first time.

But for some patients with less severe illnesses, social prescribing can actually be more effective than antidepressants. As Professor of Primary Medical Care at the University of Liverpool, Chris Dowrick is worried about the overprescription of antidepressants for mild to moderate depression. He describes a phenomenon called 'diagnosis creep' whereby people's perfectly normal reactions to serious events, such as bereavement, are then medicalised and medicated. He argues:

I can write a prescription for six weeks of gym membership as quickly as I can write a prescription for Prozac. In my own practice [instead of talking about antidepressants], I've spent a lot of time discussing approaches that the patient might have found helpful in the past, such as mindfulness, running, tai chi, or whatever.

Like many GPs, he names parkrun, which is a network of free, timed five-kilometre runs in local parks, as a prescription that 'does everything: it's very strenuous if you want it to be, it's regular exercise and it's social'.

Dowrick and other doctors aren't just thinking about how active a social prescription might make someone. There's a clue in the name: often social prescribing involves getting someone plugged in to a community and many nature- or sports-based activities do that without the need for an awkward set of introductions. There is plenty of evidence that social isolation leads to worse mental health, and conversely that feeling part of a supportive community can help people recover or alleviate their symptoms.

Once again, though, we come up against the question of money. Most doctors can generally find an activity which doesn't involve membership fees, such as parkrun, gardening or walking groups. But some sports and activities are better when you have at least a little bit of the right kit. Running, for instance, can damage your feet if you don't have the right trainers. Cold-water swimmers tend to don neoprene gloves and booties when the winter temperatures fall into single figures. My riding lessons weren't cheap. Even going for a walk in the winter requires a decent coat. Stokes-Lampard wants there to be a standard database so that GPs across the country can match their patients' circumstances with a prescription that works for them. In some cases this might require funding, in other cases the doctor can find something that is low-cost or free so that their patient needn't worry about being able to afford it.

Claire Murdoch is the National Mental Health Director of NHS England. She is also a registered mental health nurse and believes very strongly that 'drugs and therapy alone cannot bring about healing', and to that end NHS England now has a network of social prescribers who can direct people with a range of conditions, not just mental, to activities they think will help them. This can include

NHS-funded gym memberships, or personal budgets which can be spent on sports kit, or even on an assistance dog if the patient agrees with their link worker that this is what they will benefit from. There is an understandable anxiety on the part of many healthcare professionals that this spending will be written up as a ridiculously indulgent waste of money, but this underlines our overemphasis on a biomedical model when we still lack evidence that, in every single case, drugs are definitely the right course of treatment, or that the specific drugs being used are the right ones. It is hard to say what the 'right' level of antidepressant prescription should be, for instance, but anecdotal evidence from GPs suggests that these pills are often prescribed because there isn't anything else available, rather than because they are necessarily the best course of treatment.

Beyond the money that the NHS can provide, it's worth remembering how much of the great outdoors is free, and how disconnected we have chosen to be from it, regardless of how much money we have. When I presented two Radio 4 programmes on how nature and gardening can help people with serious mental health problems, I was surprised by how many people branded the act of sitting in a Bristol woodland or joining a community garden as 'middle class'. Yes, nature might be able to help, they said, but what about the people who couldn't afford to visit it? This was odd: not only are most nature reserves and woodlands entirely free to enter, they're often in city centres, or at least a short cycle or bus ride away. But nature reserves themselves can also mislead people into thinking that you have to actually travel somewhere to see nature. Even a short walk through a city centre will yield wild flowers growing in pavement cracks and on buildings. You'll also find moths, bees, butterflies and birds – not just the ubiquitous pigeon. We don't see nature around us because we have decided not to look for it, but it is always there.

Since I have started keeping my eye out for interesting flora and fauna as I go about my days, I have realised how rich life is: even inner cities have their own natural tapestry. Take Glasgow. It's not the first place in Scotland that you'd think of for hunting rare wild flowers. Yet one of my most exciting botanical finds was in a car park by the Clyde. I was walking past a messy patch of birch trees planted next to the parking spaces and, as I always do now, I glanced under the trees to see if anything interesting was growing there. It was: I could make out a series of spires with purple bells hanging down from them.

The broad-leaved helleborine, *Epipactis helleborine*, is an orchid native to the United Kingdom. It is a beautiful plant, sending up long spikes of flowers that, when you crouch down and really look at them, do bear more than a passing resemblance to the orchids we grow on our windowsills. Their petals can range from pale green to a wine-rich purple. I had spent four hours clambering over the magnificent limestone pavement at Hutton Roof in Cumbria a week before in search of these plants – but then I found them in a Glasgow car park. One of the best things about this orchid is that it doesn't just hang out at nature reserves. It is what botanists call 'gregarious'; a lovely term that suggests a sociable, outgoing plant, and which technically means a species with the tendency to grow in large groups. Being an orchid with good taste and social skills, the broad-leaved helleborine was quite understandably drawn to the weighty beauty and blunt warmth of the city of Glasgow, where it grows in vast numbers on waste ground, pavements and in car parks. It is an exquisite orchid, growing right under people's noses as they walk to work.

As I crept about between the trees, marvelling at the variety in colours in just this one population of around 100 broad-leaved helleborines, something caught my eye. Right next to a reasonably normal-looking orchid was a bright violet one. Not merely a plant with bright violet flowers, but a plant that was, from leaf to tip, completely purple. It almost glowed. I'd heard of these plants before: they have a mouthful of a name – *Epipactis helleborine var. monotropoides* – and they produce no chlorophyll at all. Instead, they get their food from a secret underground relationship with fungi.

I found that orchid while I was on a phased return to work. It was an anxious time: I endlessly feared that after a year in which I had been either on sick leave or very sick at work, I had lost my edge and reputation as a writer, that my colleagues resented or looked down on me for my inability to pull myself together, and that I would inevitably be sacked. I needed constant reassurance when I was on duty, but I also needed constant distraction from my anxious thoughts when I wasn't working. Hunting for wild flowers provided that: it was something that I enjoyed enough to become totally absorbed in. It made me excited about nature and how diverse even the flora of the United Kingdom can be. I doubt that anyone who'd seen that bright violet broad-leaved helleborine glowing away in a Glasgow car park would have left concluding that our world is dull and has already given them all the knowledge and experiences that it can. At the very least, nature can make a life made grey by mental illness seem rich again.

Self-Care: The Bad, the Ugly and the Necessary

It wasn't just rare orchids that helped me recover. Hunting for wild flowers of all sorts became an important discipline for me. I had been a keen gardener all my life, and had also spent many a childhood hour poring over wild-flower books, learning the names for coltsfoot, stitchwort and lady's smock. I already knew more about native wild flowers than any of my friends, but when I fell ill, I decided to make wild flowers an obsession to counter the painfully obsessive paranoia that was preventing me from living properly. On very dark days when the ruminations were so bad that I felt like a fly caught in a spider's web, I would still force myself out of my home in Barrow to go for a walk along the promenade opposite. It's nearly a mile long, and has dozens of wild flowers, many of them coastal specialists. I would stop at every flower, photograph it, write down its name and count how many plants there were. To the drivers of the cars whizzing by, I must have looked even madder than I actually felt, and I can't say that the perennial sow thistles and sea campions that I found cured my madness. But they stopped me feeling worse.

These sorts of daily activities are part of what is known in the mental health world as 'self-care'. This was one of the most terrifying parts of mental illness for me, as it sounded awful, like the sort of thing that people who go to spas and sit in the Jacuzzi with a glass of champagne looking pleased with themselves might do. Self-indulgent, pointless and easily ridiculed. How did this have any relevance to an illness which was keeping me away from work and making everything, from close relationships to supermarket shopping, feel like an impossible task? What would 'self-care' involve for me? Having a manicure? Buying a posh dressing gown and holding a 'girly evening' with pink Prosecco and chocolate? If this was to be part of coping with a mental illness, then mental illness was so much worse than I'd even imagined.

One mental health charity even tweeted to its followers that self-care could be laughing with friends or sitting on a swing. This really borders on the 'dance like nobody's watching' territory of memes involving sunsets and wisdom about life which generally entails being as selfish as possible.

A mental wellness industry has sprung up in recent years, too. On first glance, this could be a really welcome sign that the stigma has lifted sufficiently for it to be acceptable to buy magazines called *Happiful* or to tweet about your #selfcare regime in the same way as a beauty blogger might discuss their approach to exfoliating. That may be true, but behind some of this new culture is a dangerous misconception that mental illnesses can be cured by the simple things in life or by trying a bit harder to tick all the boxes in a regime.

At the heart of this misconception is a confusion over the difference between 'mental health' and 'mental illness'. The first is something that we all have and all need to pay attention to, just as we do with our physical health. I have no physical problems at all, save the odd self-inflicted running injury, but I still think a great deal about my physical health, making sure that I am fit, eating a balanced diet and getting enough sleep. I do have a diagnosed mental illness, but I would say that, generally, my approach to mental health is pretty good, much better than many people I know who have no mental issues at all. Our mental health can deteriorate if we are working too many hours, not sleeping enough, drinking too much, being bullied, dealing with bereavement or coming out of a miserable relationship. None of those things constitute mental illness, even though it is alarmingly common now for doctors to prescribe antidepressants to someone who is simply going through the normal emotional turmoil of grief after the death of a loved one. Grief is natural, paranoid delusions are not. That people often lump the two things together contributes to the impression that 'self-care' can solve serious illness, as well as help you keep your head while all around you are losing theirs.

It is true that some illnesses come and then go, and also that many people do find that their journey out of the acute stages of illness is made far more pleasant by cold-water swimming or their horse. But the mental wellness narrative suggests that a happy, mental-illness-free ending is always out there. For many of us, it isn't, or at least it's less round the corner and more decades away.

To suggest that running will mean you will be able to avoid relapse, or that birdwatching will stop all those suicidal thoughts that wrap themselves around you until you can't really see properly, is to lie horribly and dangerously. Because if someone does get ill again, the implication of #selfcare is that you didn't try hard enough, when all too often mental illness is as controllable as the tides.

The mental wellness industry has also contributed to the impression that the great outdoors is something for the middle class, not a free resource for anyone looking to help their mind. Hotels near my home in Cumbria now offer 'forest-bathing' minibreaks aimed at restoring your mental health – if you've got £600 spare, that is. Mindfulness retreats, 'self-care' subscription packages (all of which seem to involve an alarming amount of herbal tea) and a thousand diets suggesting that if you just read this book that tells you about the threat milk poses to your sanity, then you'll be okay: all of these things aren't just the market responding to demand as the stigma lifts. They're also a current – a rip tide, even – that risks making us drift away from what little decent understanding of mental health we currently have. Where there is uncertainty, quackery thrives, and there are few fields more uncertain than mental health.

There is also a tendency for popular mental health culture to focus on the illnesses that are more possible to fix or significantly ameliorate, such as depression, anxiety and PTSD. Even those of us with these disorders can find this frustrating, but for someone with an illness at the more severe end of the spectrum, the ignorance of what they are suffering can be, well, maddening. The *Guardian* journalist Hannah Jane Parkinson has suffered from bipolar disorder since she was thirteen, and in June 2018 she wrote a furious piece about how this new culture made her feel:

In recent years the discussion around mental health has hit the mainstream. I call it the Conversation. The Conversation is dominated by positivity and the memeification of a battle won. It isn't a bad thing that we are all talking more about mental health; it would be silly to argue otherwise. But this does not mean it is not infuriating to come home from a secure hospital, suicidal, to a bunch of celebrity awareness-raising selfies and thousands of people saying that all you need to do is ask for help – when you've been asking for help and not getting it. There is a poster in my local pharmacy that exclaims, 'Mental health can be complex – getting help doesn't have to be!' Each time I see it, I want to scream.[13]

Parkinson is rightly frustrated by the way in which mental illness can be cast as a battle to be won and then tweeted about. I have struggled with this tension myself over the past few years. I think I am right to be proud of the way I have tried to wrestle with my illness, to try to stop it robbing me of more things that are dear to me. However, that fight has become strangely easier since I accepted that I might not actually win it. In the first two years of suffering from PTSD, I was endlessly demoralised that I wasn't better yet and that I still couldn't just cope with whatever life threw at me.

For all its twee connotations, self-care *can* be an important part of walking around the black hole of mental illness. It is part of a package of treatment – and also a sign that the overall package is working well. At its most basic, self-care involves personal hygiene, decent amounts of sleep, getting dressed in the morning, eating, clearing up after yourself and so on. When well, I do these things without thinking. When I'm struggling, I have to force myself. Often when I've spiralled into a very dark place, I will look back and realise I have spent all week walking over piles of clothes, eating only cereal and not brushing my hair. These are not mad actions in and of themselves, but they're a sign that I'm leaving the physical realm because something in my mind is starting to take hold again.

Beyond those basic, essential actions is a set of activities which can alleviate symptoms to some extent. Because of the way 'self-care' has been overly commercialised by the bubble bath brigade, I'll call this 'physio for the mind' from now on. When you are recovering from an injured back, you are not just prescribed painkillers but also physiotherapy exercises. When your mind is injured, you are prescribed antidepressants, antipsychotics, lithium and so on. Those drugs are so important, but like the painkillers for the leg, they're best when they're part of a package of treatment, not the sole remedy. This book looks at how the great outdoors can form an essential part of that physio for the mind, whether it is swimming in cold water, hunting for wild flowers or walking a black dog.

But before we start jumping into those cold lakes, a word about language. You will have noticed already that I have referred to myself as 'mad', which is a pejorative term often used to stigmatise those with mental illnesses. I would never use this to describe anyone else, but it has helped me enormously to separate out what is a symptom of my illness from that which is an intrinsic part of my personality. To be able to say that something was 'mad' is a huge comfort to me, because I then do not end up sinking deep into the mud of guilt that follows particularly bad bouts of illness. I still apologise to my friends and family for certain incidents, just as I might had I vomited all over them. But I know that my madness is no more my fault than a stomach bug would be. So, to me, the word 'madness' has become a kindness. This book, I hope, will at least give anyone with any mental illness some more ideas about how they could offer the same kindness to themselves.

CHAPTER TWO

Sowing the Seeds of Sanity

There aren't many reasons to celebrate the era of lunatic asylums. People were chained up, away from their families, experimented upon and used as entertainment. The Bethlem Royal Hospital in London became famous under the nickname of 'Bedlam', a place where rich, fortunate types would turn up to watch the patients. Hogarth depicted these events as being like a freak show, a sightseeing spectacle, rather than a compassionate visit designed to enliven the inmates' lives and raise money for the hospital. Beer and nuts were sold to visitors as they enjoyed the suffering of those being treated in front of them. But among the misery and mocking were some glimmers of good sense: many institutions for the mentally ill also had gardens designed to help the patients.

Thomas Prichard was the superintendent at Abington Abbey in the 1860s. He wrote that 'the care of the gardens being, in many instance entrusted to patients, serves as a double purpose – of affording wholesome occupation, and of promoting a tranquil and cheerful tone of thought'.[1] Gardening was part of a patient's daily routine: the Middlesex Asylum allotments were tended by the patients and the produce from those plots was taken from an 'asylum dock' to market for sale. Asylum gardens themselves were beautiful and some of the country's best-known designers such as William Goldring were behind their creation.

Inpatient treatment has changed dramatically in this country, but the gardens remain at many of the hospitals. Even those that have moved site still try to set up new gardening plots for their patients because they recognise the benefits that horticulture can bring, even to those who may spend the majority of their lives in a hospital.

The Bethlem Royal Hospital, now part of the South London and Maudsley NHS Foundation Trust, has extraordinarily beautiful grounds. Its 270 acres of green space include orchards, meadows and bluebell woods. It also has a walled kitchen garden run by its occupational health team.

When I visit, on a sharp April morning, the orchards and wall-trained fruit trees are heavy with blossom and everyone I meet is keen to emphasise how very sick you have to be to end up a Bethlem inpatient. This is not somewhere that people with manageable mental health problems spend time. Many of the units house 'forensic patients' – the health service term for someone who has been through the criminal justice system – and are locked, with towering fences around the outdoor exercise areas. The site itself is beautiful, but it has a sad quietness to it, as you'd expect from a hospital trying to look after so many people with serious mental health problems.

Peter O'Hare, the head of Bethlem's Occupational Therapy team, explains that many patients are so very ill when they first arrive on the wards that any kind of strenuous activity is out of the question. Some have severe anxiety disorders which may mean that just leaving their ward is something they'll spend many weeks working up to. Others have phobias involving germs, which means the garden is both a terrifying prospect and an important part of their treatment as they prepare for the outside world. The hospital also treats people with eating disorders, who normally have the opposite problem: they are desperate to get outside and exercise, but can only do so once they are gaining weight and engaging with their therapy.

As a measure of quite how unwell the people deemed well enough to enter the garden still are, all the tools are locked in metal cages and counted in and out at the start of each session. A wooden pergola, made by patients in the hospital's therapeutic woodwork classes, has been specially designed to collapse if someone tries to hang themselves on it. String is used sparingly for the same reason.

All of these precautions are subtle, though. The garden feels like any other. It has a beautiful greenhouse with a voluptuous grapefruit tree at one end, and rows and rows of seed trays with pumpkins, tomatoes and flowers popping up. Pear trees and soft fruit like the Japanese wineberry and loganberry are trained neatly against the red brick wall. Raised beds – all made by patients – have young lettuce plants popping up. Primroses throng around the wildlife pond and two huge rosemary bushes are in full bloom by the locked gate. O'Hare says that many patients respond particularly well to the sensory aspects of gardening, and that the rosemary bushes are part of a series of beds deliberately planted with this in mind. There are long rows of lavender, herbs and plants with particularly tactile leaves, like lamb's tongue, which has silver-green woolly leaves just asking to be stroked.

Why do touch, smell and taste help a psychiatric inpatient, I wonder. O'Hare says it's a way of grounding someone, of taking them away from whatever is raging in their mind and forcing them to notice something that's actually happening at that very moment. For that reason, mindfulness classes often start in the sensory garden, as they help patients refocus for the session ahead.

Many of Bethlem's inpatients are on site for a good long time. Some of them are moving from the high-security prison Broadmoor through different levels of secure accommodation at Bethlem, which can take months or years. These patients are the ones who often gain the most from the garden, says O'Hare, as they have a chance to invest in it and see the fruits – apples, pears, apricots and so on – of their work.

Julia Durbin is tidying the workshop after its latest group when I wander in. She's a horticultural therapist and is buzzing after a conversation with one of the patients. He told her that he wasn't sure about the garden when he first set foot in it, but it has made such a difference to his time at Bethlem, and it is even helping him engage with his therapy better. Durbin argues that gardening has a clear impact on how well patients respond to the more formal aspects of their treatment, such as psychotherapy and medication. She also observes physical changes in someone's demeanour after just an hour on the plot:

> You see someone come in all hunched up, and after a while their shoulders relax. Or else they won't want to work with other people and will be in their own corner of the garden, but will end up gravitating towards the rest of the group as the sessions go on.

Gardeners generally say they love the long-term nature of the hobby the most. You have to wait months between sowing a pumpkin seed and harvesting its fruit, and those months are busy with feeding, watering and protecting it from pests. Seeing young plants mature to the stage where they start producing a harvest is satisfying for anyone, but even more so if you are in hospital without a great deal to do. Boredom is a huge problem on inpatient wards, which is why psychiatric hospitals have a reputation for being smoke-filled: cigarettes help pass the time when you're waiting to be well. But Bethlem has recently gone smoke-free (or as smoke-free as possible: wandering around the grounds, I find a bench out of the way where patients clearly sneak for a quick smoke). The hospital's management decided that it wasn't right to be allowing people whose physical health is often far from where it should be to damage their lungs with cigarettes. Unlike cigarettes, the garden doesn't just give patients something to do, it also helps them improve their physical health.

A Bit of Earth

Bethlem is by no means the only psychiatric hospital to use gardens as part of its treatment. All over the world, mental health inpatients are prescribed gardening by their doctors. In Singapore, some hospitals have been designed so that plants are visible throughout. Its Institute of Mental Health has won national horticulture awards for its patient gardens. There's the Friendship Garden, which has around thirty patients visiting the plot each day to work with plants and exercise in the outdoors. Its dementia patients were growing agitated when they couldn't get outside, and so it created a therapeutic garden for the geriatric-psychiatry wards. Its programme to treat psychosis early on includes gardening, and patients have views from their ward windows of greenery too, such is the emphasis on the healing power of plants.

In New York, an agency called The Bridge helps rehabilitate and house people with mental health and substance abuse problems. As part of this support, it has an urban farming and horticulture programme which has six gardens across the city, including one on the roof of its clinical headquarters in Manhattan. They grow fruit and vegetables which they then use in workshops on healthy eating and in meals for clients. And those taking part often end up getting jobs and more qualifications in horticulture. The Chicago Botanic Garden is open to the public and is part of the worldwide work on plant science, but it also has a horticultural therapy department which runs sessions for people with a range of mental health problems and special needs in its carefully designed Buehler

Enabling Garden. The focus is on improving people's mental health through teaching them to take a cutting from a plant which they can then take home, using flowers and leaves to make works of art, and planting seeds. Their team also visits treatment centres to work with patients there.

Even gardeners who have never experienced mental health problems will readily tell you that they don't just grow because they want a smart garden, or cut flowers, or their own fruit and veg. They garden because the very act itself is good for the soul, even if that soul has never been troubled by ill health.

I have gardened all my life. When I was six, my mother gave me my own 'patch' in the garden. My planting choices were eccentric: a miniature Christmas tree joined some strawberry plants, a buddleia, a pumpkin (which didn't make it to fruiting) and two huge clumps of asters and marguerites. I was very rarely present as a child, spending most of my time either in a book or constructing an elaborate imaginative world. In my mind, my patch was in fact an island, and I dried the stems of the asters and wove them into hurdle fences and rope walkways between the sturdier plants for the inhabitants to get around in. Buddleia leaves folded in two and joined with a grassy rope became boats. I would spend entire weekends tending to my patch, weaving invisible worlds as I did.

My childhood was a very content one, and my time in the garden the happiest of all. As a teenager, I spent six months off school with a post-viral fatigue, and ended up swaddled in a duvet on the sofa, either watching gardening programmes on daytime TV or poring over my parents' copies of D. G. Hessayon's Garden Expert series. By my mid-adolescence, I was unusual in knowing the common and Latin names of most garden plants by sight, and was constantly trying to take over the planning of our new back garden. I spent spring and summer evenings after school weeding the heavy clay borders, and planting more cultivars of buddleia than my parents had even known existed. I tried to start a wild-flower patch at the far end of the garden, persuading my father not to mow the lawn there, and secretly planting snake's head fritillaries among the turf. These plants mesmerised me then, and still do now. They have a chessboard pattern on their petals which seems impossibly unnatural. The flowers are deep or light purple, or pure white, and they naturalise in damp meadows.

Our garden, newly reclaimed from grazing pasture, was perfect: the clay was either sodden or baked so hard that a drill would have been better than a spade during the summer. The damp grass became home to cow parsley and lady's smock, a lilac-coloured spring wild flower that comes into bloom at that time of the year when the evenings are not cold but cool and dewy, and the blackbirds sang thoughtfully well into the gloaming. Teenagers spend a great deal of time thinking about their feelings, but still struggle to articulate what's really going on. I would never have been able to say, aged fifteen, that the thing that made me happiest was being out in the garden. But given I was always finding more excuses to be outside with plants, I had clearly found something that made me feel more content than anything else.

When I lived in flats with no outdoor space at all, I found myself restless, yearning for that 'bit of earth' that Mary Lennox asks for in *The Secret Garden*. I covered a second-floor balcony in one flat with plants, growing kale and salad leaves. When I was offered an allotment in a village four miles away from my home, I caught the bus with a spade in a camping rucksack on my back. I planted rows and rows of raspberries and other cane fruit. I dug out two huge beds for pumpkins and squashes, and grew so many that I was still eating the final stored fruits as I sowed the seeds for the next season. My allotment site was a quiet one: it was often just me and an elderly fellow who was the third generation to garden the same plot. We swapped tips – and later in the year, courgettes, which is something gardeners don't do to be kind and generous but to get rid of the endless supply of these vegetables. But we largely gardened in silence. It was just us and the red kites that circle over the Chilterns.

I had never thought about gardening more deeply than that I loved it. I never realised that the methodical act of pruning my apple tree or moving from bed to bed pulling up weeds was something that helps soothe people's minds. Or that the satisfaction of planting a tiny, dry seed and seeing it turn into a monstrous sunflower with leaves so big you could shelter under them during a burst of rain might be good for mental well-being. To me, it was something I had to do, because when I didn't, I didn't feel as happy.

It seems almost too obvious and common sense that gardening makes you feel good. It's such a popular hobby, and so many people swear by their allotments or back gardens as remedies for their minds, whether they've spent their life in and out of a psychiatric ward, or they just have tricky days at work from time to time. There are famous gardeners who see plants as essential to their mental well-being, too: Monty Don is the presenter of *Gardener's World* and author of countless books on the subject. In 2019, he argued in an article for *Gardener's World Magazine* that gardening could become as serious a treatment for mental illness as the pills that doctors prescribe:

> Gardening makes you feel good. There are lots of ways that this works. As a depressive, I know that just going outside does some good. If you have a garden then the rewards are there. The flowering of the rose you pruned or a lettuce you grew from seed or a robin singing just for you. These are small things, but healing in a way that medicine tries to mimic.[2]

I know now that even a session sorting out my compost heap can make me feel more alert and calm. I've thinned the young fruits on my espalier apple tree as an explicit way of calming myself down from a panic attack: the slow search for the tiny apples, and the methodical act of pinching them off their stems turned into a soothing rhythm for me, and by the end, both I and the apple tree felt lighter.

What is it about gardening that helps so many people? Clinicians are so used to seeing their inpatients using gardens that it's surprising there isn't more research backing up what has for centuries been a widely-held hunch. Many studies have found that gardening leads to a significant reduction in symptoms of anxiety and depression, an improvement in mood, self-esteem, attention span, sleep and physical health. It is understood that activities such as gardening, knitting or drawing stimulate lower-frequency brain waves which help us relax and think creatively. And, as we already know, there's an outdoor bonus to be added to any mindful activity: knitting is indeed very relaxing, but with the soft fascination of the outdoors, gardening can be even better. One Bristol-based academic found a bacterium in the soil called *Mycobacterium vaccae* could cause the brain to release serotonin.[3]

But we do not know, for instance, how long-lasting the effects of gardening are: a 2013 review concluded that 'at present there is… insufficient evidence that relatively brief gardening-based interventions can have long-term effects for people experiencing mental health difficulties'.[4] A King's Fund report in 2016 complained that there were not enough randomised controlled trials to prove the cause-and-effect of gardening for mental health, but it did add that 'many observational and qualitative studies are consistent with a wide range of health impacts across mental and physical health behaviours'.[5]

Many gardeners running mental-health-focused projects report that certain plants seem to help more than others. There are those with particularly strong sensory qualities, such as herbs which give off strong fragrances. Rosemary, sage, thyme, mint and lavender are all reasonably hardy perennial herbs which don't need a great deal of work. We all know how useful they are in the kitchen, but they're also marvellous at grounding someone who is outside and working in the garden. There's nothing wrong with breaking a few young leaves off these plants and chewing them while you work, as well as enjoying the smell that their foliage emits, particularly on warm evenings when the essential oils start to move in the air.

Texture, too, is an underrated but important part of a sensory garden. The lamb's tongue in the Bethlem garden is one example of a plant that just feels really good. Succulents like houseleeks are rigid and fleshy, while fuchsia flowers are ever so satisfying to squeeze when in bud, so that the bloom pops open like a botanical jack-in-a-box. Feathery, fluffy grasses like *Pennisetum villosum* are perfect for running your hands through, and you can rest your palms against trees with interesting bark, like birch, snake-bark maple and eucalyptus. Sound is often neglected in gardens, or drowned out by some discordant and annoying wind chimes. But plants like bamboo rustle against one another in the wind, birds visit feeders and berry-laden bushes, and leaves crackle underfoot. Sound can often be a challenge for people with acute mental health problems, as it adds to the roar inside their heads. In a garden, though, the slow, gentle sounds of nature can help to calm that roar.

It's easy to assume that sight is simple to cater for in a garden. After all, anything green and growing is easy on the eye, given humans have evolved to relax around plants. But what about the winter months, when there isn't much green to be seen? Plants with bright barks like dogwood and willow will stop a sensory garden from being grey and sad in the dormant months. There are three main colours of dogwood: yellow, orange and red. The most vibrant cultivar is *Cornus* 'Midwinter Fire', which ranges from flame orange to deep red to bright yellow. Planted in a group, this shrub looks stunning from a distance and up close. Even better when it has a backdrop of a deep green evergreen shrub, like box, yew or holly. Willows have an even greater range of colours, including green, purple and another bright fiery orange. Both dogwood and willow are very low-maintenance. Every March, you should prune the branches down to a few inches above the ground so that new, fresh, bright ones grow in their stead. I tend to prune my plants in thirds, so that I still have a few available to add colour and structure to the garden while the younger ones are emerging. And the pruned branches make very good supports in the garden, particularly for vegetables like peas. Just be careful not to let the willow sprout and turn your entire plot into a thicket.

Allotments

As with all of the therapeutic activities we'll explore in this book, everyone needs a different dose of gardening. Some need supervised inpatient gardening programmes which last for the very long time that they spend in hospital. Others are best suited to pottering around on their own plot. Some only discover how good gardening is by accident.

Tracey Crouch is Conservative MP for Chatham and Aylesford, and signed up for an allotment with her partner Steve when he was off sick from work for nine months, having lost his voice. As a radio presenter, this meant he couldn't work, even though he was clinically well in every other respect. An allotment seemed a good way of keeping him busy while he waited to be able to speak again. 'He was going a bit potty,' says Tracey. 'We got it to help support his mental health and well-being. It kept him active and gave him something to do.' The plot had been abandoned, and the couple spent their first year clearing it and planting as much as they possibly could. They weren't gardeners, and were surprised to discover that by the end of that growing season, they'd managed to get a decent harvest.

Tracey came to see the allotment as a place to look after her own mental health. She has spoken out about her anxiety, and works in a high-pressure and often dysfunctional world. Being split between

Westminster and her constituency means she only gets to work at the allotment every few weeks, where she has a 'binge' of weeding, planting and harvesting. And whenever she has a chance to do one of those binges, she finds herself calming down. As she explains:

> It's a place of peace and serenity. Even though it is by a busy road, you just feel so far away from everyone when you are down there weeding out carrots and onions. Then you're not thinking about Brexit. It is such a nice place to go and get absorbed by the surroundings.

> I was down there a few weeks ago on one of my morning binges, and it was raining and spitting, and then the sun [would come out again], so I was running into the shed, working in there, then running out again as soon as it was dry. You're there, face to face with the seasons, and that's really nice to be part of that.

Annabelle Padwick also uses her allotment and towpath garden as part of her efforts to tackle her anxiety. She was in her twenties, struggling to leave the house and had limited access to mental health support. Her allotment represented a happy, halfway house between staying indoors and the daunting wider world. She found the process of growing vegetables so absorbing and satisfying that she now credits her allotment with saving her mental health alongside psychotherapy, and has set up a non-profit organisation and support network called Life at No.27, named after the plot. The organisation provides gardening and well-being therapy for struggling children and adults. Her allotment therapy sites enable GPs to prescribe gardening as an alternative therapy for adults and she delivers programmes directly into schools for students in need.

She is also beginning to offer a buddy system for people who want to start gardening for their mental health, but don't want or have their own space. They can learn from more experienced gardeners on a regular day and time, which provides new friendship and consistency. It also means that growing your own veg doesn't turn into a stressful experience involving a lot of wilted plants.

A few years ago, allotments became incredibly trendy in the UK – much like wild swimming is now. You couldn't move for articles about how having an allotment was the best thing you could possibly do. As a result, everyone, even those who didn't really like gardening, signed up for one with their local authority, and waiting lists soared so that it would take decades to reach the top and get your own bit of earth. The demand has reduced a little in some areas now, but waiting lists remain lengthy in many parts of the UK – and some local authorities have started to close sites and sell the land for development, thus restricting the availability of plots still further.

This doesn't mean that people without their own back yard or local allotment cannot grow, though. As well as the therapeutic community gardening projects like those at Bethlem and in cities around the world, there are many public gardening projects springing up all over the UK, particularly in urban areas where many people don't even have space for a wheelie bin, let alone some plants. Once again, these community gardens don't just give people a chance to get dirt under their fingernails, but also a chance to build relationships. The Incredible Edible network of gardens is one example: in Bristol alone, there are forty gardens including urban allotments and veg beds on station platforms. It isn't run as a mental health project, but many of its participants, including its Bristol founder Sara Venn, are adamant that without gardening, their mental illnesses would be much harder to manage.

Community gardens can be the first line of mental health treatment for groups that do not traditionally engage with formal health services. In Fresno, California, there are state-funded community gardens for refugees and immigrants who tend to be more isolated, less able to afford healthcare and less likely to find a therapist who understands their culture. They are also much better for those who cannot commit to the level of work that a personal allotment needs (which is quite a lot, and if it's not near your home, then just getting there can feel like a real chore if you're not enjoying the constant battle with weeds).

And you don't even need a stand-alone plot to set up a community garden. London has a reputation in the rest of the UK for being an unfriendly city. People are often moving between neighbourhoods, staying for only a couple of years at most, and it's hard to put down real community roots. But another project in the capital showed that sometimes neighbours just need a reason to get together. In *Veg Street*, Naomi Schillinger tells a story of how her Islington neighbourhood burst into bloom when residents started growing vegetables in their front gardens and sowing flower seeds in tree pits. Schillinger and a neighbour, Nicolette, then signed up fifty households to take part in a growbag scheme. They held events where people got to know each other, and gradually the plants started to take over the neighbourhood. 'It's no exaggeration to say that our project has transformed the feel of the neighbourhood,' Schillinger writes.[6]

New York has a similar bustle to it and, aside from Central Park, it's not known for being a garden city. But some gardeners have seen bits of earth where others have just seen traffic islands, derelict properties and empty plots. In the 1970s, a group of guerrilla gardeners started planting sunflowers on the empty land in the centre of roads, placing flower boxes on the sills of abandoned buildings and 'seed bombing' empty lots. They started setting up community gardens on empty land, and moved from a band of gardeners working on the edge to a non-profit organisation which works with the local authorities and helps gardening groups set up their own plots for growing fruit and veg. Guerrilla gardening is a worldwide movement of people who either don't have their own space for growing plants or are fed up with the grey urban landscape around them and want to make things prettier for everyone. It can cause problems in areas with established native ecosystems, though, and it's worth making sure that you aren't 'seed bombing' an area with truly native wild flowers, as this doesn't help anyone. But on a forgotten traffic island or flowerbed filled with nothing other than discarded drinks cans, guerrilla gardening can make the surrounding environment – and therefore everyone's mental health – a little better.

Peer out of the window of any suburban train and you'll end up feeling rather dismayed by how few people do anything with their back gardens. Some can't manage them because of health problems, and there have been attempts to matchmake between these owners of neglected plots and the people desperate to garden. For a few years, a UK network called Landshare tried to match plotless gardeners with people who were unable to manage their back gardens. Once again, this didn't just help satisfy itchy green fingers, but it also allowed relationships to grow between often isolated elderly or disabled people and the keen green types who signed an agreement to look after their land. However, it sadly closed in 2016 after struggling to support its website. There are local landshare schemes still in place in some areas, but wouldn't it be powerful if the cause was taken up by social prescribers? The NHS deals with many people struggling to stay in their homes because they can no longer manage them or who are weighed down by crushing daily loneliness. At the same time, it sees many people with mental illnesses who could use gardening to manage some of their symptoms. In some cases there might be safeguarding considerations, either for the gardener or the garden owner. But this is why the involvement of a social prescriber would be so powerful, as they would have far better resources and knowledge than volunteers on a badly-supported website.

The Great Indoors

Even though there are initiatives that work with people to overcome physical barriers to gardening, there are those whose mix of illnesses prevents them from getting out into a garden. Some of us have weeks when leaving the house is just very hard. Even though I am a sociable type, when I am unwell I can feel terribly frightened of the outside world. I often feel like a peeled egg, with no shell protecting me. Sometimes I know that staying indoors will just be gentler than trying to force myself outside. I'm mostly lucky, though: I tend to find the pull of the outdoors to be stronger than the force of my illness. But this isn't the case for everyone.

The wonderful thing about plants is that their sheer inventiveness and entrepreneurial spirit means that if you can't go to the garden, the garden can come to you. Houseplants were, for a while, generally limited to a grouchy-looking spider plant on an elderly woman's fridge or a dying orchid on a work desk. Now, they're fashionable enough to be the sort of thing that people who call themselves 'Instagram influencers' take an interest in, posting stripped-back photos of their variegated *Monstera deliciosa* plants and boasting about reaching the top of a waiting list for a fiddle-leaf fig. Once again, plants have an extraordinary ability to work their way into our minds and make us go a little loopy. Even those of us unbothered by plant trends can gain a great deal from growing indoors. You can still stimulate your mind by learning about how to care for those plants – the same methodical activities of watering, pruning, deadheading and tidying still apply under a roof.

Once again, the research on houseplants and mental health isn't particularly definitive. One review published in the *Journal of Environmental Psychology* found the presence of potted plants led to lower stress levels and less discomfort among people in a variety of hospital settings.[7] Another study found men appeared to relax when tending to plants in an office environment.[8] But other than general research on plants in the workplace and hospital settings, there isn't much on whether houseplants at home can help your mental well-being, and how much of a difference they can make.

Of course, plants can be a source of stress, too, if they regularly end up shrivelled and brown on a windowsill. People often give up on indoor gardening because they think they're good at killing plants. This might indeed be because they really have forgotten to water something for six months or have watered it so much that it has rotted all the way through. But more often than not, it's either because the plant just isn't in the right situation (too much sun, not enough sun; burned from the bottom up on a radiator; frozen on a draughty windowsill) or because it was damaged in the shop. Many supermarkets sell their houseplants right by the main doors, which means delicate specimens like orchids end up getting a nasty – and often deadly – blast of cold air every time someone walks in. Sometimes this is due to thoughtlessness, but sometimes it's because plants that die easily mean a customer will come back and spend more money on another poor specimen. It's best to decide that a plant casualty is someone else's fault and find something that suits your home better. There are plants that are really very difficult indeed to kill, such as *Sansevieria*, or 'mother-in-law's tongue'. Climbing, heart-shaped plants such as *Philodendron* and *Pothos* are very happy in low light, while cacti prefer it if you forget about them. And the best thing about houseplants is that you have to try very hard indeed to get weeds growing among them. They're often far less work than an outdoor garden and can soften the lines of your home.

It's Not Just About Plants

It would be a mistake, though, to assume that it's the act of gardening itself that provides all the benefits. In fact, some people whose lives have been turned around by working in gardens aren't particularly bothered by plants. John Wetherell is one such case: he insists that while he likes gardening, he's never really caught the bug. But it was working in a garden that changed his life.

John has been sectioned twice, with a diagnosis of paranoid schizophrenia. He was rough sleeping for over a decade, and came across horticultural therapy when peering at the noticeboard in a homeless hostel. He ended up being referred to Thrive, the best-known horticultural therapy charity in Britain, where he worked once a week in the Battersea Park Herb Garden. According to his horticultural therapist Richard Jones, John's well-being noticeably improved when he was handed responsibility for the planting of one of the larger beds in the Herb Garden. As John said, it gave him the agency to make decisions for himself:

> I knew I was happy in the garden. I had expected some kind of regime of psychotherapy, but the benefits turned out to lie in the social aspect. I'd been so severely isolated I didn't have any social skills at all. But here it didn't matter: the garden is a great leveller. You can talk to anyone if you're weeding together.

Thrive helps its clients gain horticultural skills and, where appropriate, return to the workplace. But in John's case, a day's one-off admin volunteering led to him getting an office job within the charity itself. While John feels our spiritual connection to nature is hugely important, it was the job that transformed his life.

He is self-effacing, claiming that his social skills are still not quite there, but over a cup of tea in a north London cafe, I enjoy talking to him so much that I fail to notice the time – something that doesn't often happen when I'm with allegedly socially adept politicians. He's pleasantly blunt, too, which leads to him telling me that my question about how gardening has improved the symptoms of his mental illness is 'irrelevant'. I had been so preoccupied with the effect that methodically sowing broad beans had on someone's mental state that I had barely acknowledged the social aspects of gardening. Thanks to the Thrive garden, John now feels a part of society in a way he hasn't for decades.

Thrive doesn't just help people with mental health problems, but those with physical and learning disabilities, stroke and heart disease patients, people with dementia and those who are visually impaired. It started out in 1978 as the Society for Horticultural Therapy and Rural Training and its founder Chris Underhill was inspired to set it up after seeing the way gardening helped people who were blind or had learning disabilities when he was doing voluntary service in Africa. He advised hospitals on how to use their land to help their patients, and encouraged a more disciplined approach to gardening which involved wearing the right clothes, using the right tools and working the land in the best way to ensure plants grew well. The charity now has centres in Berkshire, London and Birmingham. It helps around 1000 people a year, and 94 per cent of its gardeners say they feel better after attending Thrive. Perhaps more striking than how people feel is how they then behave as a result of the gardening therapy they receive. The charity set up a garden in the back yard of homelessness hostel Hopkinson House. It included a greenhouse and raised beds, and residents learned to garden and cook with the produce they'd grown. The hostel managers noticed a decrease in substance misuse and improvements in overall well-being as a direct result of the garden project.

Damien Newman runs the Social and Therapeutic Horticulture training programmes at Thrive today. He says that the charity places an emphasis on three important 'therapeutic opportunities' in its programmes: time in nature, social interaction and meaningful activity and occupation. 'Different people engaging in our programmes experience and self-report this in different ways,' he adds. 'Some will talk about friendship, others enjoying gardening, but in general anecdotally they reference all three.'

So gardening isn't just a therapy because time with plants is healing. It's what gardeners experience when they are with one another that can also make a difference. Many horticultural therapy projects are run on the basis that their clients will need help for quite a long time. This isn't about a few weeks of sowing sunflower seeds, but many years of working in a garden. Of course, that suits the pace at which gardens grow: sowing seeds might feel nice, but it isn't a patch on watching the seedling emerge, spending weeks protecting it and then planting it out in an open bed. Months of work and patience reward you with a sunflower. Years of working in the same garden means you can harvest apples from the tree you planted and pruned. Newly-planted beds change their character over time, plants scrambling into one another and creating colour and texture combinations you'd never dreamed of doing yourself. Gardens aren't supposed to be quick fixes. Often, that's also the case for recovering from mental illnesses.

In Sheffield, the Greenfingers allotment project set up by Support Arts Gardening Education (SAGE) has been running since 1998, and works with some of the most socially excluded mentally ill people in society. Clients often attend for years. It covers five large allotments with raised beds, a polytunnel, a greenhouse and a big shed with its own basic cooking facilities. It was set up by a local GP surgery after doctors there found that its disadvantaged patients weren't keen on the mental health services that were available to them. SAGE Greenfingers offers a light touch for people who need therapeutic horticulture.

As with the work that Thrive does, the therapeutic horticulture at SAGE Greenfingers doesn't involve talking about your past while pruning a rose bush. It isn't therapy; it is an activity with therapeutic benefits, which is an important distinction. For them, the way to help improve their clients' lives is the gardening itself, rather than a formal talking therapy. The project follows those five ways to mental well-being: connect with others, be active, keep learning, give to others and be mindful. Louisa is the service manager and explains that:

> … participation in the gardening groups provides our members with the opportunity to experience all of these things. People can keep coming to the groups as long as they need to, and people stay with us for months and sometimes years. We also have a very low staff turnover and the workers supporting our groups have been with us for years [too]. This leads to trusting relationships building up, consistent support, and other group members are able, over time, to offer peer support.
>
> It is the gardening, alongside being within a safe environment and within a familiar group and supported by caring and consistent workers, that provides the therapy. We do not offer counselling or any other therapeutic intervention other than social therapeutic horticulture.

It's clear that it's not just the act of gardening or any other nature-based activity that helps. It's also the people you're with who help you break out of isolation, and repair lost social skills and confidence.

What gardening does is make all of those rather daunting things like working on self-esteem seem much more manageable. The soft fascination offered by an outdoor environment full of the scent of herbs, the sensation of soil between the fingers and the sound of birds busy in the bushes around the plot has the same effect on a mind struggling to learn to build relationships as an outdoor setting has on a runner struggling to keep going. It doesn't make it simple. But it makes it much less unpleasant. The runner on a treadmill can only focus on the thud-thud of their feet and the latest rolling news on the big screen in front of them. The person in the therapy room can only focus on the fact that they are there for therapy because all manner of things seem to have gone wrong. Being outside and noticing other things takes away a little of that discomfort. The great outdoors is a free mental analgesia.

CHAPTER THREE

Obsessing About Nature

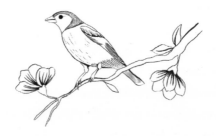

'Isabel, I never thought I'd say this to anyone,' said a politician, 'but you need to get out less.' He was teasing me after discovering that my weekend plans, in the middle of the coldest winter we'd had in a while, were to go and sit by a river for several hours, hoping a kingfisher might turn up. The snow kept on coming that winter, but I just put on more and more layers (including two, sometimes three, pairs of gloves) and trudged outside.

I had learned that getting outdoors to obsess about nature was crucial to my staying sane. It replaced the more conventional 'self-care' techniques that everyone had been advocating to me, and had helped me to manage my illness to the extent that I was able to come off sick leave and return to work.

One of those conventional techniques was mindfulness. I admit that I struggled even to understand the concept. At first, it sounded to me like the frustrating bit in a yoga class when the teacher tells you to spend ten minutes focusing on the spaces in your togetherness, and all you really do is start remembering that you left wet washing in the machine and then find yourself wondering why you've paid so much money to sit in a studio worrying about your domestic chores.

The man who popularised mindfulness, Jon Kabat-Zinn, describes it as 'paying attention in a particular way, on purpose, in the present moment, and non-judgementally'.[1] Eh? This both makes no sense and also sounds as off-putting as those silent yoga classes.

Perhaps another one of Kabat-Zinn's drops of wisdom will help: 'It is remarkable,' he writes, 'how liberating it feels to be able to see that our thoughts are just thoughts and that they are not our "reality".' Aha. Now we are getting somewhere. The difference between our thoughts and the present reality is so important in managing mental illness. When we realise how out of step what is going on in our mind is with what is actually happening around us, then we have a real chance of stopping those thoughts from taking over.

Mindfulness isn't something you'll only find in a yoga studio or some kind of spiritual healing workshop. It has entered the mainstream, with the National Institute for Health and Care Excellence (NICE) in the UK recommending it as a means of preventing depression in patients who have had three or more bouts of the illness in the past. Schools are offering it to their pupils. Prisons are running 'mind/body workout groups'. Never ones to be left behind, even trendy companies like Google now have mindfulness. There's even a mindfulness group in the staid old Houses of Parliament.

Of course, when you start to burrow down into the research, you find a lot of conclusions calling for 'more work' on who can really benefit from the technique and who can't, but the Oxford Mindfulness Centre has found that something called 'mindfulness-based cognitive therapy' (MBCT) can be as effective at reducing the recurrence of depression as antidepressants for people who have experienced three or more episodes of the illness.[2] The University of Surrey conducted a randomised controlled trial into an online mindfulness course which found a 63 per cent decrease in depression, a 58 per cent reduction in anxiety and a 40 per cent reduction in perceived stress among those who took part – and this effect was still there three and then six months later.[3] Another trial involving the same online course found a 25 per cent decrease in rumination (more on this shortly), a 26 per cent reduction in fatigue and a 33 per cent improvement in sleep quality.

The Mental Health Foundation investigated the benefits of mindfulness in 2010 and reported neuroscientific studies finding that the brains of people who regularly practise mindfulness have differences in the areas associated with decision-making, attention and awareness, and that the left prefrontal cortex, which is associated with positive emotions, is more active.[4] The practice has also been found to reduce the severity of symptoms during a depressive episode, to help people with bipolar disorder who have a high suicide risk, to improve the symptoms of generalised anxiety disorder, and to reduce depression in older people on a long-term basis. It also works as a preventative treatment for people who have not had any mental health problems.

Even grizzled MPs who attended the mindfulness classes in Parliament were impressed. One told the Mindfulness All-Party Parliamentary Group: 'I found the ethos, thinking and practice totally compelling and, additionally, free of "psycho-babble", religion and spiritual allusions. A very, very enriching experience.' Another said: 'The mindfulness breathing techniques and practical exercises have helped me to cope much better with the stresses and strains of a highly demanding job and gain a better work–life balance.'[5]

Nevertheless, I could never really get to grips with the biggest mental health trend of the last decade. Everyone, from my psychiatrist to my friends who've battled mental health problems, recommended it. I'm sure to people who like lying still, it's great, but I am a fidgeter and I resented my sessions. I felt guilty about missing them, but they really didn't seem to make any difference to my state of mind. Sometimes they even made things worse, as I struggled to block out thoughts that I'd spent all day wrestling with, only to invite them through the open door with ten minutes of sitting in silence.

I don't bother with those sessions now, not because I'm not looking after myself properly, but because I've found a better way of being mindful than lying on the floor, twitching resentfully about having to spend another ten minutes going nowhere. Now, I use botany as my mindfulness – and it works.

Outdoor Mindfulness

I have already described my sick mind as a personal 'torture chamber', and the most terrifying instrument in that chamber is not the one that stops sentences forming, or even the one that makes me think it would be better for everyone if I disappeared. It is the one that makes the ludicrous seem totally, terrifyingly real.

Many people imagine that obsessions and paranoid delusions are always of the sort that the film *A Beautiful Mind* depicted: government plots, secret codes and so on. To someone without the mental illness that creates these terrors, they seem laughable. But to the owner of the mind in which they whizz around, they are as real as that festering washing that you forgot to take out of the machine.

But my own obsessive worries were less exotic. They involved two totally terrifying fixations. The first was that my partner was on the brink of leaving me. Every single day. The other was that I was about to be sacked from my job.

I was the youngest ever Political Journalist of the Year. I was one of the two writers who drove the most subscribers to the *Spectator*, the magazine I worked on, and yet every day I was convinced that my colleagues wanted me gone or that my boss saw no value in continuing to employ me. I was able to write pieces about the government's policymaking process and Theresa May's judgement in managing her Cabinet, but when it came to my own life, I could not determine what was real. I needed to be able to train myself to discern the difference between the terrors invented by my subtle, clever, manipulative illness and reality.

This is the real value of mindfulness: it takes you out of your mad mind and refocuses you on what is actually in front of you, hence the wishy-washy-sounding stuff about the present moment. It's just that for me sitting still in a room doesn't really help me focus on the present. In fact, it offers an even quieter space for the mad thoughts to make themselves heard. So how could I do what I needed to do?

I hadn't realised that it was possible to use nature as my own mindfulness exercise until I came across Kevin Widdowson. Kevin has worked for various different wildlife trusts over the past decade, and therefore knows how much of a difference nature can make in people's lives. His favourite projects are those that involve showing people – whether toddlers or pensioners – a little of the rich diversity of the natural world. But nature isn't just important to Kevin because it's his livelihood. It is also vital to his mental well-being.

Kevin has recurrent depressive disorder, and cannot remember a year from his adolescence onwards without at least one depressive episode that's lasted longer than a month. He has had spells in hospital, and continues to need therapy and medication. But nature is also one of his treatments:

I deliberately use wild flowers for my mental well-being. It's part of my cognitive behavioural therapy: my therapist and I have built it into my programme to give me the techniques for mindfulness, distraction, the use of analytical thinking and even using it as an analogy for mental health.

Initially my therapist was saying that when I was walking around town I should notice signs, shop windows and so on, but that's not interesting to me. I also tried CDs on mindful meditations but they would tell me to imagine I was in a forest, and the description of the forest wouldn't be what I know of a British woodland. It just made me want to be in a real wood, rather than imagining one. When my therapist got to know me a little better, he realised that we could tailor the mindful walking to my love of botany.

I'll be walking, noticing the plants and noticing the trees, and trying to do the grasses too. That process of noticing things as I am walking along, it's really mindful and it's about keeping yourself in the present.

I then need some way of bringing that indoors, so I will collect samples of plants appropriately and I will bring them home to analyse them after my walk. This has become a ritual for me. I'll get my microscope, my hand lens, my botanical keys out. The tactile side of this, the feel of my copy of *The Wild Flower Key* by Francis Rose… it's an old friend that I get comfort from.

Winter is a challenge for botanists, as there are fewer flowers. But Kevin has taken to identifying trees by their twigs and bark, and plants through their vegetative characteristics or fruits. He has a pot of around ninety twigs in his house, and tries to identify as many of them as possible. And that way, his mindfulness doesn't lie fallow during the colder months.

Kevin has long had a problem with self-esteem, which isn't a mental illness in itself but which can lead to or exacerbate certain conditions. As he analyses the plants he's found, he writes cribs on how to identify them, which he shares with others on Facebook and Twitter. And seeing how his knowledge is encouraging and teaching others helps improve his sense of self-worth. Kevin describes this as 'showing off', but it's not, really; it's sharing your delight in what you've found and what you know with other people so that they have a chance to experience that for themselves. His own treatment for his mental health problems helps other people see the world in finer detail, and therefore appreciate it more, too. Mindful botany is a routine that helps Kevin leave behind the thoughts that his illness forces on him, recognising them as unreal and refocusing him on what is real, which is the richness of nature.

I also find that a walk outside is a powerful way to focus on the present. Wherever I am, there is so much that is obviously real and obviously good: the proud, big yellow flower heads of the perennial sow-thistle, *Sonchus arvensis*, the tiny teeth on the tepals of a broad-leaved dock, *Rumex obtusifolius*, or a pair of jays arguing noisily on a wall until one storms off in a flurry of brown and brilliant blue (the Latin name for a jay is *Garrulus glandarius*, which fits this bird's noisy, garrulous character). Outside, around nature, my mad thoughts are so much more easily identified as mad, just as a perennial sow-thistle is easily identified by its height and the golden glandular hairs on its confident, regal body. Identifying plants using their defining characteristics is not a million miles from the discipline of identifying a mad thought by its own special features. And one of those special features of the mad thought, *Insana sententia*, is that it has no connection to the present reality. For this discipline to work, you do really need to try to do a mindful activity every day. It is like building a muscle: you can't expect to have strong triceps after just one session in the gym.

So I've dropped the guided meditation apps and instead have tried to have at least fifteen minutes in every day when I just go for a walk outside. Sometimes this is a walk along the street in central London or through St James's Park, which is handily right next to the House of Commons, where I am often loitering. Sometimes I hop off my bike on my morning commute and spend ten minutes on Barnes Common or on a scrappy patch by the river, looking for wild flowers and giving my mind the space that other people manage to get from a recording telling them to lie down and close their eyes. The methodical act of looking for plants stops my mind from whizzing into a long rumination about something unhelpful. The satisfaction of finding a plant, whether it be a common dock or a surprise rare chlorotic orchid, lifts my spirits just a little, and those fifteen minutes with no bustle, talking or worrying helps even a tough day feel a little bit more manageable. Categorising plants helps me put my mind in a little better order than it was before. A messy mind is no good on busy days: it's as unhelpful as a messy handbag when you're desperately trying to find your front door keys so you can rush inside and out of a downpour. I now don't find it hard to incorporate those fifteen minutes into even a frantic day because I save time by having a healthier mind that can bounce from task to task and solve problems and tricky characters just a little bit quicker.

Here's an example of one fifteen-minute walk that I did while writing this book. One day, while in Edinburgh, I set off into some nearby woodlands (when you start looking, you'll realise that there are local nature reserves even in cities), and turned my phone on to airplane mode. My focus was on noticing everything around me: the delicate spiced smell of fallen leaves; the corky feel of a spruce bark or the marble-smooth trunk that lurks behind the spiky leaves of a holly; viburnum berries; white dead-nettles in flower; the way beech leaves in autumn turn from green to hammered copper and gold; sycamore roots gripping on to an outcrop of black sandstone. I haven't told my mind to behave in the way it does, but the rhythm of looking at the world around me slows it down and helps it swing ever so gently from thoughts about the things that are bothering me, because, ah, there's a group of mushrooms on a rotting log over there or a coppiced rowan which is so old and gnarled that it forms a bridge over the woodland floor.

Woodlands, as we will see later, do have a special effect on the soul. But these mindful walks don't need to be anywhere particularly picturesque. On another fifteen-minute walk in a very grey bit of London, I found much that was green and alive. There were tiny little bumps of green growing in the cracks in the pavement, which look on first glance to be moss but are in fact flowering plants called procumbent pearlwort, *Sagina procumbens*. A close look, if you don't mind squatting down on the pavement and whipping out a hand lens in full view of the passing traffic, reveals tiny, pale green flowers with either tiny or totally absent petals. Then there are the liverworts, which also love a good crack in the pavement. Strange, flat, flappy little things that they are, the liverworts don't reproduce through seed but spores. The part of the plant that produces the spores looks just like little palm trees on a desert island. Even if you don't fancy looking like an oddball by peering at the pavement cracks, just knowing and noticing that there is treasure at your feet wherever you are can feel quite satisfying.

Then there are the tough street plants. They know how to look out for themselves in an unwelcoming world. Groundsel, smooth sow-thistle and knotgrass are the sort of wild plants that no one cares about, but which happily go about their business without any praise or attention. In my garden, I would pull them all up as soon as they appeared, but on the street, I feel a strange respect for their tenacity in finding just enough grime and dust to be able to eke out a living between pavement and building. There are also the kerb creepers, the plants that choose to live between pavement and road. Another one of my favourites is the pineapple weed, *Matricaria discoidea*, which grows on field margins but also in urban hinterlands like gutters and kerbs. This looks like a daisy that left its petals at home by mistake, as it only has a central green cone, which looks a bit like a pineapple, as a flower. It's not just that this rather modest daisy doesn't mind living in places that other plants would turn their noses up at, it's that the pineapple weed also smells of pineapple when you pick it and crush it gently between your fingers.

City tree pits are another botanical treat, and my favourite plant that likes to lurk there is the gallant soldier. Such a magnificent name for a member of the daisy family that also appears to be missing some of the white petals on its small flowers. But gallant soldier is actually a corruption of its Latin name *Galinsoga*, which is one of those pointless facts that nevertheless is quite nice to know. Gallant soldier has a relative, too, called shaggy soldier, a rather hairier character which has a few other tiny defining features that you can only really spot when you've got your hand lens out. The two plants like to sit around on the streets like soldiers who have returned from war and fallen upon hard times, but nevertheless are still as tough as their military boots in their ability to thrive where no one invited them.

Learning what these plants are, and the stories behind their common names, provides me with another important technique for dealing with mental illness: distraction. Mindfulness may form part of the daily stretches that you do to prevent mental pain, but the truth is that even when you are diligent, your illness can be craftier and will sometimes outwit you. Alternatively, events might make it harder for you to stay on top of your mind. And this is where obsessing about nature comes in handy.

We're Going on an Orchid Hunt

The madness of Orchidelirium sounded far more fun than the one that was keeping me from the job I loved on my second bout of sick leave in 2017, and so I decided to give it a go. I drove a little way to a nature reserve which I knew had a few different species of these plants, and started hunting.

Latterbarrow Nature Reserve is near Witherslack, Cumbria, and is a quiet, secret mix of meadow and woodland. It didn't take me long to find my first orchid: there was a greater butterfly orchid, *Platanthera chlorantha*, just a few steps into the meadow. These are quite easy to spot, unlike some of the other members of the family. They are over thirty centimetres tall, with a good number of white to pale green flowers which have two petals shaped like wings, and a long spur like an insect's body. That was my first find, but the treasure hunt at Latterbarrow absorbed me for three hours. I found common spotted orchids, *Dactylorhiza fuchsii*, and an early purple orchid, *Orchis mascula*, hiding under some trees, the spring sunlight illuminating it quite smartly.

There's a special hit that you get when you're flower-hunting, especially for unusual plants or ones that, like orchids, have a special cultural cachet. Orchidelirium isn't so much an obsession as an addiction, but it's one that leaves me feeling quite a bit stronger and calmer, even on days when my mind is trying its best to be bad. Firstly, you have to get your eye in so that you have a chance of spotting some species. Your common spotteds, early purples and greater butterflies are all very well as you can see them at the other side of a meadow. But some of their family members are a little more coy. This means you have to be completely fixated on the ground in front of you and, even then, you can overlook a specimen. Such concentration is naturally a distraction from the mad stuff that's trying to get your attention, and as it is eventually rewarded with a discovery, it's easy for your mind to start latching on to it as an enjoyable habit.

My first proper discovery was the common twayblade, *Neottia ovata*. This is a quiet plant that really seems to want to hide from the attention that many of its relatives make such a play for. It was growing at the side of a path in the woodland, its green flowering spike trying as hard as it could to blend in and look normal. The individual flowers do have that orchid look about them, with a long forked tongue hanging down. When I tried to find it again later, as I made my way back to the car, it took me half an hour of peering hopelessly at the ivy, wild garlic leaves and other distracting foliage on the woodland floor before I could make it out again. By this point the mad thoughts were barely registering, so determined was I to find that dratted flower.

The second tricky orchid was the one I'd come to Latterbarrow specifically to find. The fly orchid, *Ophrys insectifera*, actually tricks wasps, not just with its shape but also the texture and smell of its flowers. While the poor insect is pounding away at the entomological equivalent of an inflatable sex dummy (though plants are better at making these seem realistic than humans will ever be), the fly orchid is dropping pollen on to the unsuspecting wasp's back. Those insects might find themselves irresistibly drawn to the fly orchid, but I found it so hard to find that I nearly gave up. Eventually, I sat down in a patch of the meadow and stared around, trying to refocus my eyes once again to look at the minute details of flowering grasses until, finally, the fifteen-centimetre-high orchid started to emerge from the undergrowth like one of those Magic Eye pictures. It really is a curious plant, and while I hope one day to recover from my mental illness, I will never lose my wonder at how clever nature is that a flower can slowly evolve until it is able to deceive a wasp. That wonder does make life a little richer, especially when it's not until you're thirty-one that you discover a fly orchid exists at all, let alone how it works.

I have realised that I will never get to the end of the plant kingdom. There is always more to learn, more to excite my curiosity. Knowledge is power in so many ways, but knowledge for its own delight seems particularly powerful when you are mentally ill because it is such a simple way of reminding your sick mind that there is so much of the world that is worth exploring.

In that summer of sick leave, I visited the lady's-slipper orchid, *Cypripedium calceolus*, and spent four hours hunting for dune helleborines, *Epipactis dunensis*, at Sandscale Haws National Nature Reserve in Barrow-in-Furness. I eventually found those helleborines with a close relative, the green-flowered helleborine, *Epipactis phyllanthes*, hiding cheekily under some willows at the top of one of the biggest dunes in the reserve. As well as snapping photos of the flowers themselves, I took a happy, flushed selfie of me next to them to send to my friends.

'Was it worth it?' asked one pal who had been following my adventures all day. 'Actually, I can see it was. You look much happier than you've seemed for weeks.'

That happiness hit didn't cure my depression, and it only lasted a little while. But it added up to help make a sick day feel a little less of a waste because I had achieved something in finding a new species and learned more about how diverse our flora is. It also helped alleviate the symptoms by taking my mind away, even for just a few hours, from the thoughts that left me wanting to turn myself off entirely.

The effect that wild-flower hunting had on me during such a difficult time was infectious. A friend who also suffers with sometimes debilitating depression decided to copy me, even though she hadn't grown up poring over flower books as I had. At first, I would receive pictures of common poppies, along with hesitant messages asking for their names. Within a few months, though, Katie was starting to help her own friends identify common flowers. 'On one level, it gives me a task,' she explains. 'I like tasks, and I like learning. It makes me appreciate where I am, and as the flowers are often in grotty places it teaches me to look for the good in the rough.' She, too, enjoys finding pineapple weed growing in strange places. 'It makes me notice. [It] takes my mind off turmoil and has really helped me when I've had that awful, head-collapsing torture when I just want the ground to swallow me up.'

Katie also loves sharing her new knowledge with friends. After she learned what an orangey-red-flowered member of the *Asteraceae* family was, she showed a picture of it to a friend. The plant was fox and cubs, *Pilosella aurantiaca*, and it reminded her pal of the fox and cubs flowers he'd seen in his own childhood. So many of us have old emotional connections to plants that we've forgotten.

I started sharing what I found during my 'fifteen-minute nature fix', as I called it, on Twitter each day. This kept me honest: there was more of an incentive to make sure I'd taken those fifteen minutes. It also prolonged the effects of each fix, as there is something very cheering about sharing things that have made you even momentarily happy, like the lumpen shape of some of the grafted cherry trees in St James's Park, for instance.

It was all the more satisfying when I discovered that my tweets about tree bark and pavement weeds had led people I'd never even met to try mindfulness outdoors. Miriam is a student who contacted me to say that a nature fix is 'one of the best things I've ever done':

I've had quite bad anxiety for a few years now. I've been seeing a therapist and trying loads of different techniques, including mindfulness apps, all those things, but none of them had worked. I personally found the apps useless but the fact that so many people were recommending them even though they didn't work for me actually made me more stressed.

But with the nature fix, even though it's only fifteen minutes each day, it's fifteen minutes purely to myself, not thinking about work or relationships. I get fresh air and realise the world isn't too bad after all. When I would have really bad periods of anxiety, I would not see anyone. I'd skip lunch and go and work in a separate room but now at least I'm getting outside a bit every day and recollecting myself. I have found that it makes me a generally happier and more positive person. Perhaps it's realising that the world still goes on, or that there are beautiful or incredible things within it.

It was Kevin who taught me the value of the regular nature fix which I then passed on to others like Miriam, and though it was a couple of years before we then met, I'd credit him with being one of the biggest factors in my recovery. I would never have managed to get back to work or learn to control my mind if I had stuck to the mindfulness apps. In fact, while I still prefer to do a nature-based mindfulness session every day, I have built up sufficient mental muscle to be able to use those apps and find them helpful.

From time to time I do try to exceed that fifteen-minute fix. I don't have weeks of sick leave yawning ahead of me for Orchidelirium these days, but I still try to organise a proper hunt for one rare flower or another once every fortnight. That satisfaction of really immersing myself in the natural world helps me, whatever my mental state at the time.

When I am aware that my mad thoughts are taking up more of my attention than they deserve, I have developed a botanical strategy for turning down the volume on them. It came about after reading *The Orchid Hunter* by Leif Bersweden, a lovely tale of an eighteen-year-old who decides to spend his pre-university gap year trying to see all the fifty-two different native orchids that grow in this country. I read Bersweden's book during the 2017 political party conference season. Party conferences are relentlessly busy weeks inside windowless conference centres with people who hate one another, but I love them. The problem with the 2017 season was that it marked a year since I had become so seriously mentally ill that I had needed sedation, and had left the Tory conference in Birmingham early to start my period of long-term sick leave. I was quite obviously better this time around, but I was still nervous that the same thing might happen again.

I needed something to distract me and calm my mind, and *The Orchid Hunter*, which bounces from fly orchids to lady's-slippers to autumn lady's tresses, did just that. It wasn't just that this teenager was so delighted by the weirdness of nature, but that his enthusiasm was so infectious that I wanted to plan my own orchid hunts so that I too could see the lizard orchid, which apparently looks like a reptile, but smells like a billy goat.

I started plotting good orchid sites on a map, and found the act so immersive that I now do it whenever I notice the warning signs that my mental state is deteriorating. Working out those warning signs is a really important part of self-care. These can be very subtle changes, such as a sudden thudding feeling of total exhaustion, or my shoulders becoming so painfully tight that I can't turn my head properly, or me starting to look for the 'evidence' that my partner is about to leave me, or that some other mad catastrophe is looming. With the help of my therapist, I wrote out a list of early and late warning signs that I need to keep an eye out for.

Once I notice that there's a red light on my dashboard, I take a few minutes to work on my orchid plan. I read books, apps, blogs, tweets – whatever is available at the time – and try to find more potential sites for a certain orchid, before saving it on a special

'Orchid Hunt' list on Google Maps. One of my favourite parts of my orchid hunt planning is to work out where in Glasgow might be particularly good to find more broad-leaved helleborines, as it involves combing planning applications, botanical databases and local blogs. Perhaps this is more satisfying for me than it is for other people, given a basic part of my skillset as a journalist is researching and combing lengthy documents for a single important nugget of information. But then again, who doesn't like a treasure hunt? Either way, my orchid hunt reminds me how little of our native flora and rich habitats – even city car parks – I have so far seen, and helps me plan ahead for the future, thus reminding me that life is worth continuing with. This gives me a sense of purpose and is a very simple way of looking forward to the future.

For the Birds

One afternoon, I popped into the London Wetland Centre, which I'd heard had broad-leaved helleborines in flower. Most people come here for the birds, so the woman at the reception desk was a bit baffled when I asked her if she knew where in the large network of boardwalks and marshlands the orchids were growing. Eventually, I found them, and once again had to explain to passing birders why I was crouched in the undergrowth without a flying creature in sight.

One of those birders was chatty, and I ended up telling him about my orchid-hunting exploits. He swapped stories with me about the rare birds he'd seen, including there at the Centre on the outskirts of London. As I listened to him talk, I realised that though I knew so little about birds, we were speaking the same language and in the same tone: we were both gaining an enormous but quiet satisfaction from being quite alone, watching and hunting for nature. Birds move, plants stay where they are, but as we hunted for our different prey, we used the same techniques: getting your eye in, then learning about the defining characteristics of different species so that, over time, it gets easier to tell a godwit from a long-tailed tit without even seeming to think about it. I have no idea if my birdwatching friend had a mental health problem, but I realised that it's not just plants that are powerful; nature has a strong hold over our minds, however it manifests itself.

In his memoir of how the great outdoors helped him recover from a mental breakdown, the writer Richard Mabey says his psychiatrist was 'always trying to persuade me to take myself up into the hills' of the Chilterns where the author lived. He writes: 'He'd seen me once after I'd been roaming there for a while among the red kites, and glimpsed, I think, the person I'd once been, and what the birds had symbolised for me.'[6]

Red kites are fine birds, with five-foot wingspans and a way of coming down to earth that resembles a fighter jet corkscrewing its way down to the ground. Mabey isn't the only person to have found the sight of them soaring around and around on the thermals above the Chilterns totally mesmerising. And he also isn't the only person whose mental health improved so visibly after seeing birds that even his psychiatrist offered to drive him there to see the kites again.

Joe Harkness is one of the most vocal advocates for the benefits of birdwatching for mental health. He has written a moving book called *Bird Therapy* which follows his birding adventures, which he took up after having a nervous breakdown and a diagnosis of obsessive-compulsive disorder (OCD). He has tried to take his own life a number of times. 'I've had problems with alcohol and class A drugs and I smoked a lot of cannabis when I was young. It wasn't until I had this particular breakdown that everything was sorted out for me,' he explains. It was only when Joe had his breakdown that he realised that nature could actually help him manage those obsessive thoughts: 'When I had my breakdown I was just going for a walk. I had just started taking a medium dose of sertraline, which felt like the effect of coming up on class A drugs and it was freaking me out a bit.' He saw and immediately recognised a buzzard as it flew over his head. It reminded him of times with his grandad, who would show him wild birds on walks. Joe started to realise that being outside and seeing birds like buzzards, great crested grebes and kestrels helped his state of mind. Joe's dose of sertraline and counselling have made a big difference to his illness. But so has his birdwatching:

> When you look through binoculars or a scope, you are cocooned in those barrels or in that tube and the entire focus of your mind or vision goes on that. It's the ultimate focused meditation. You could be anywhere, looking at a woodlark, and nothing else matters at that particular moment because everything else is blocked out.

He also tried twitching, which differs from birdwatching in that it is all about the thrill of chasing across the country to see a particular rare bird that has turned up. It is not uncommon for twitchers to travel from Land's End to John o'Groats to see two particularly interesting birds. It's also difficult to find anyone who says twitching helps with their mental health. Indeed, it seems to hinder it. 'It was just horrific,' says Joe. 'I could see how it could take over your life.' It is possible for anything good to become a harmful way of opting out from society or numbing mental pain without solving it. Perhaps the occasional twitch of an interesting bird might work well as part of the normal routine of watching all the birds that come and go on your local patch. But when something becomes an obsession that gets in the way of life and relationships, it's probably not all that handy as a tool in a mental health kit.

Paul Brook is another person who finds that birds make things a little better. He works in communications, and has suffered from depression and anxiety for a decade. The illness tends to affect him in dips, and Paul takes antidepressants and has had cognitive behavioural therapy (CBT) as well. His counsellor suggested he should try to make regular time for an interest of his, which for Paul was birdwatching. During a period of sick leave, he started forcing himself to go out looking for birds every day, and then tried to go for a short walk in his lunch breaks once he was back at work. Even though he had young children at the time, Paul made time for the birds, 'pushing the buggy and trying to look around rather than down, then looking up to see what was flying over'. He also loves watching the birds on the feeder in his garden:

> We have started to notice the different behaviours of the common birds that visit. We have a wren which [always] comes into the garden in the same way. It starts on the fence on the left-hand side of the garden, it hops along a few steps and then it drops down into a bush. It's always the same bush, and then it goes off to the back fence and flies off somewhere. It's kind of taken on its own little character.

The way Paul speaks reminds me of the fondness in the voice of Kevin Widdowson, who taught me about mindful botany, as he described the routine of going through his wild flower books to identify specimens. It's not just his 'childish excitement' when he sees something rare, but the comfort of a routine that has very little to do with work and family. Even his favourite bird, the yellowhammer, reminds him of his childhood, as well as looking rather lovely:

> I like the colour yellow, it's happy and warm and it's something I associate with when I was growing up and we would walk the dog down a country lane, where the yellowhammers used to sing. They've got a very distinctive call as well: [it sounds like] 'little bit of bread and no cheese', and I have a lot of empathy with that because I hate cheese.

Hiding from Loneliness

One day, inspired by my bird-loving interviewees, I went back to the Wetland Centre, but this time not for the orchids. It was a bone-cold day, and not the friendliest start to birdwatching. I walked into a hide, which is a small, sparse-furnished shed with narrow horizontal windows for birders to peer out of with their binoculars and lenses, and wooden benches to perch on. Even in there, sheltered from the wind, my fingers were too cold to really work. But along with the cold, I also found a strange sacred peace in that chilly room. Birders moved in and out in reverent silence. When they spoke, it was in a low prayerful murmur.

'Anything of interest?'

'Saw a redpoll by the WWF hide. There's a jack snipe over there by the marsh grass just now.'

'Oh yes, I see him. Seen the bittern?'

Everyone seemed to be murmuring about this bittern. I had no idea what it, or any of the other birds they mentioned, looked like. Soon enough, I made a friend.

'Anything interesting?' she asked.

I explained that this was my first time brandishing binoculars and asked for some tips. One of the very best things about naturalists is the way they cannot contain their enthusiasm. It is the opposite of impertinent to ask them what they've found and how they found it. My new friend was just like that: she turned on her camera and showed me a shot of a pert little bird with a smart feather darting out at the back of its head. 'This is a lapwing,' she explained. 'It has lovely iridescent plumage.' Then she gave me some advice on which hide would give me the best chance of finding it, and trudged off, swaddled against the cold. I saw a lapwing shortly afterwards, and went home feeling rather pleased with myself.

I had expected birdwatching to feel like a cold version of botany. And in many ways it was. There was the same need to stay vigilant, which I noticed as I considered how I had barely thought about anything other than the birds whose names I didn't know. There was the discipline of looking for distinguishing features, albeit plumage rather than petals, before thumbing through a bird book to find what on earth I'd spotted. Then there was the satisfaction of discovering that I'd found a shoveler, which is a rather natty duck with a very practical-looking beak. But there are differences, and good ones, too. I thought I'd developed patience enough during my four-hour-long dune helleborine hunt. But birdwatching requires a whole new order of unflappability, because instead of feeling as though you are still achieving something by striding around a lot, you have to sit still and hope that something may turn up. And finally, in that watchful, cold silence, I have learned to sit still with my thoughts.

One of the principles of mindfulness is learning to recognise that unpleasant thoughts have somehow pitched up in your mind but then deciding to let them go, rather than letting them pull you into the swamp of insanity. A healthy mind is rather like a wetland reserve, with all sorts of thoughts flitting around, alighting briefly, and then flying off again. A sick mind latches on to negative thoughts and turns them over and over for hours, rarely moving from the spot where they landed. I found these ruminations some of the worst symptoms of my illness. Their regular interruptions meant I could not concentrate on work. I doubt I would have been able to regain the natural flight pattern of my mind without medication and therapy. But I doubt that those would have worked had I not learned to coax my brain on to healthier ground using nature.

Sitting in a bird hide is far less terrifying than lying on my own floor, staring at the ceiling. That's because, while the monastic simplicity of the hide leaves me quite alone with my thoughts, what is going on outside the open wooden hatch means those thoughts have less hope of taking hold. After all, I might miss a bittern.

On my second visit to the Wetland Centre, I could tell something interesting had turned up when the calm started to stir. The long line of birders (all about thirty years older than me, and all men wearing green coats) began to move more quickly, to pass on instructions and then to call out, 'There it is! Right in front of the Hedley hide!'

I'd never met any of these birders before. I had listened quietly as they'd debated whether one bird was actually a Mediterranean gull, or whether they were 'just talking ourselves into it'. But, all of a sudden, I was being ushered across the hide to a telescope so 'the young lady can see her first bittern'. I didn't even know how to use the scope but I peered gingerly into it.

And there, camouflaged like a tiger against the reeds, was this bittern that everyone had been murmuring about. It looked, to me, like a heron that was pretending to be a python, with a much fatter and snakier neck than its relative. These birds were causing such a stir because they have long been scarce, falling to below a dozen in the UK, before conservation efforts started to turn things around.

By this point, I needed to return somewhere warmer, and toddled back to the cafe. The room was buzzing with birders, cheeks rosy, fingers still lily-white with cold, all swapping stories of the dunlin, the sparrowhawk and, of course, the bittern. Most of the birders were again men, which didn't exactly contradict my own preconceptions of the hobby as something men did to get out from under their wives' feet on a Saturday. But there were couples wandering around, too: mostly of retirement age and so clearly comfortable in their gentle discussions about whether it was a pochard or a tufted duck hybrid that they were both peering at. Botanising has generally been a solitary hobby for me, but I found that not only did I rather envy these couples who murmured about murmurations, but I also enjoyed the quiet companionship of the hide.

Depression often makes us shut ourselves away from the world because we fear we have nothing interesting to say and that we won't cope very well with the company of people. When I am particularly unwell, my natural inclination is to cancel seeing friends and family, even though a bit of quiet company never makes me any worse. A bird hide feels like a good halfway house: you can get outside and be in your own company, but you find yourself being slowly reminded of the joys of other people, as they help you find the bittern and you help them find the snipe.

So, birdwatching now forms a slightly different part of my mental health toolkit. It's handy in winter when I've had my fill of identifying plants by their skeletons or leaf rosettes. It's also a gentle way of reminding me not to hide from people when I am feeling fragile, and of keeping my mind healthy through learning.

There is plenty of research suggesting that learning is a good way of looking after your mind. It might sound odd, given most adults regard learning as something that stops in your early twenties once you've graduated from university. A 2011 study by the Mental Health Foundation of adult education courses found that, on average, participants with mild to moderate depression and anxiety had improved by the end of their course. Their diagnosis on average shifted from moderate to mild, and a number of them found employment afterwards.[7]

Learning opens up new adventures. The more I learned about birds, the more I wanted to see a kingfisher. I'd only once seen a bright blue line along a river which I presumed was a kingfisher in flight. But that was all, and I couldn't stop thinking about how magnificently-coloured these birds are.

I bought a book on kingfishers and started following various photographers on Instagram who made it their business to watch these shy birds. Kingfishers spend their whole lives by rivers, hunting fish with extraordinary precision. Despite their flamboyant colouring, though, they don't like attention, and will shoot off at the slightest movement from the riverbank. This was going to be a challenge. I couldn't just pitch up in a hide and expect one to turn up. I needed to work at this, and working at it turned out to be just what my mind needed, too.

Over the following months, I researched where kingfishers liked to hang out near my home. I discovered a great deal about my local area: the River Wandle, for instance, has many kingfishers living along it. The Duke of Northumberland's River in Twickenham was just down the road from me, but I'd never heard of it before. It wasn't just a lovely, quiet kingfisher habitat, but it also had a fascinating history: this river was man-made in Tudor times to supply nearby mills. Once again, I was distracting my mind with the richness of the world around me, even in the less salubrious areas that both rivers bubble through.

One spot on the Wandle turned out to be particularly good for kingfishers. There was at least one breeding pair, and a local photographer kindly let me perch in the hide that he had created on the riverbank. This was no London Wetland Centre hide, though: it was a hollow under an elder tree, hidden from the kingfishers' view by a camouflage net. I spent two days sitting on that river, listening to the birds sounding their whistley hoots as they whizzed up and down the water. I realised that I couldn't fiddle with my phone or become too distracted by my own thoughts because the kingfishers' fishing visits were only seconds long. One of the best opportunities I had to photograph a bird came when I was briefly checking my emails. I heard a 'plop' from the river water, looked up and there was a male, whizzing away again, fish in beak. From then on, I focused totally on the water in front of me.

The local photographer, Guy, visited me one evening and told me how much work he had put into getting his shots. It had taken him months before he managed even one passable photo of a kingfisher. The first few weeks were spent walking up and down the river to work out where the birds were most likely to be fishing. Then, he spent months removing brambles from the riverbank so that he had a quiet cubby in which to hide. 'I've gone a whole month without getting a single photo,' he told me. He's down by the Wandle most days, and has even named the birds he knows well. His favourite is called 'Ziggy'.

I could tell that 'kingfishing' kept Guy going in some way. 'Sometimes I'll realise I've been sitting on this bank for hours, without thinking about anything,' he said. I wanted that feeling too: when I am particularly unwell, I just want to be able to turn my mind off. Waiting for these fascinating birds seemed like a particularly good way of doing just that.

Sometimes, though, illness can grip too tightly and we find ourselves stuck at home. Or, we can't afford to pay for a camera or membership of a wetland centre. But the wonderful thing about birds is that they turn up without you asking and without you paying. Yes, you can travel to a reserve and enjoy the sacred quiet of the bird hide. But don't ever forget that, even in central London or the noisiest bits of Birmingham, there are wonderful creatures flying overhead. It might be a chance sighting of a rare bird like the rather shy but wonderful woodcock in your local park. Or it might be the birds in the garden behind your home that doesn't even belong to you.

As a student I used to love listening to the thoughtful sound of a blackbird singing in my next-door neighbour's garden on dewy May evenings while I procrastinated over essays. I still rejoice when the days warm up and the wood pigeons coo endlessly from the fresh green trees. Wood pigeons also have a marvellous flight pattern. They flap like mad to get their plump bodies airborne, then soar, clearly imagining they look just like a raptor on a thermal air current. Then, with a shock, they realise they are, in fact, just like Buzz Lightyear and are no longer flying, but falling with style. So they start flapping frantically again to pull themselves out of the dive they've fallen into.

In the summer, the birds are on the nest or have migrated elsewhere. Birders start to migrate themselves, on to dragonflies and damselflies, just as botanists find themselves examining lichen in midwinter. One day at Foulshaw Moss Nature Reserve in Cumbria, back on sick leave after a relapse, I saw a man peering excitedly at the reeds.

'Seen anything of interest?' I asked, now practised in the language of naturalists.

'There're white-faced darters here,' he said. 'A little way back from the water is where I've seen them.'

I had no idea what these were, but they turned out to be rare dragonflies, recently reintroduced. They did have white faces, and gentle spots on their lacy wings. I found a pair in a mating ring a few minutes later.

Before bothering to look at the insects, I had noticed only the flowers of the bog cottongrass and the sparkling, dangerous leaves of the carnivorous sundew plant. Now, I saw azure damselflies lowering their mates into the water to lay eggs, then pulling them out again, and large reds resting on the boardwalks. Later, one landed on my shoulder. There's a line in Alice Oswald's beautiful poem 'Dart', which charts the course of the river through the voices of people living and working along it. A naturalist the poet meets near the source says:

> I let time go as slow as moss, I stand
> and try to get the dragonflies to land
> their gypsy-coloured engines on my hand.[8]

There is no end to the natural world, which means that each one of us can make our minds move as slow as moss as many times as we need. And as for moss, well, that's just another thing to start obsessing about.

Counting the Snowdrops

When it comes to obsessions, though, it's hard to beat Galanthomania. Like the Orchidelirium of previous generations, this fixation can drive people to spend absurd amounts of money on tiny bulbs. And, like orchids, snowdrops have played an instrumental part in helping me deal with my madness. They might be some of the smallest plants in the garden, but snowdrops have a strange cult of collectors around them who are willing to pay hundreds of pounds for just one bulb if it's from a plant with slightly different features. The tiny differences between the green markings on a snowdrop petal can drive up prices just as 'Tulipmania' did in the Dutch Golden Age. Every February as these flowers come into bloom, so do the eBay sellers, hawking rare varieties which are distinctive because they have a yellow marking on their petals or ovaries, rather than the more common green one, or because that marking has mutated to look like a frowny face, as with Galanthus 'Grumpy'. The bids can soar into four figures for particularly sought-after snowdrops. The irony, of course, is that to appreciate these tiny yet expensive differences, you have to kneel down on the ground and peer rather closely at the flowers – at precisely the time of year when kneeling on the ground is least pleasant.

What drives that obsessive behaviour? Well, it's a darn sight healthier than many other obsessive behaviours, and if you struggle as I do with obsessive patterns of thinking, you may find it helpful to start collecting something that interests you (though your bank manager may steer you away from snowdrops). It's also the emotional pull of these plants. They are the first flower to bloom in winter. And they are so, so dainty and well known that so many of us remember being shown them by our parents and grandparents when we were little. There are memories in snowdrops, as well as promises about the future.

I have avoided full snowdrop mania: the most I have spent on a single snowdrop bulb is £40 for 'Lady Elphinstone', a double-flowered yellow form which looks like a ballerina's tutu. The reason I even spent that much on one tiny plant is that snowdrops are a symbol that I use when I am having a particularly rough time. These plants appear just at the time of year when it seems as though January is going to go on for the rest of your life, when your feet are often both wet and freezing, and when your days involve getting up and going home in the dark, with perhaps a brief glance at the sky from your office window every so often. They are a sign that the dark days are going to end, but they also manifest beauty during the dark days.

In fact, there is strong evidence that noticing little signs of hope every day can help rewire your brain so that you are less likely to focus on negatives the whole time. You see, our brains are so incredibly complex (and, for many readers of this book, miserably complicated) that it is possible to retrain them in the same way as someone might learn a new physical skill requiring different muscles. This ability to change the way your brain responds to things is called 'neuroplasticity'; a posh way, perhaps, of saying that it is, in fact, possible to teach an old dog new tricks. It's worth knowing about if you struggle with depressive thoughts as retraining your brain can make such thoughts a little easier to bear.

One of the best known neuroplasticity exercises involves gratitude. Now, I know that immediately a section of readers are starting to tune out, expecting something twee that would irritate them more than help them. But bear with me: there is some good research behind it, and ways of expressing gratitude that don't make you feel like a mug. There are various studies showing that making a daily or weekly list of things to feel grateful for increases your well-being.[9] Why is this? Researchers from the National Institutes of Health in the United States discovered that people who were thinking grateful thoughts had higher levels of blood flow in the hypothalamus, which is the part of the brain that regulates a lot of our key functions like body temperature, sleep, hunger and stress.[10]

The potential of the great outdoors for improving neuroplasticity, and therefore alleviating some of the symptoms of mental illness, goes far beyond plants. There are many studies demonstrating the links between exercise and improved brain plasticity.[11] A 2017 study of people with major depressive disorder (MDD) found that exercise not only improved mood among those with MDD, but also had the potential to improve neural efficiency.[12]

There are plenty of pop neuroscience and psychology books out there which now claim that you can rewire your brain and fight depression using exercises like listing five things to be grateful for each day. There's clearly a big demand from people who would like their minds to be less negative, to forget the insults and to have a few more depression-free days, but the claims are often oversold. Our neural pathways are not the only factors at play in mental illness, and it would be irresponsible to claim that a gratitude journal is going to change your life. But the evidence so far at least suggests that it might help.

For a while, I tried writing down three good things from each day. It was helpful, as even at the end of a hard day, I could still think of the kindness someone had shown me or even something as simple as the satisfaction of a warm drink in cold weather. But the practice also forced me to think back through my day, which wasn't always particularly satisfying. Often, I would find that while I was grateful for the things on my list, I would also end up thinking a great deal more about the bad bits of the day which I had just reminded myself of by doing the exercise. Perhaps unsurprisingly, I stopped doing it.

Once again, though, nature has an answer. Professor Miles Richardson, who leads the Nature Connectedness Research Group at the University of Derby, decided to test an alternative to gratitude journaling as part of his work on nature connectedness. He asked fifty people to note three good things in nature each day for five days, and a control group of forty-two people to note three normal good things in their day. 'We found the three good things in nature much more effective than the basic three good things,' he says. The nature group became more connected to the world around them, and this led to improvements in their psychological health. 'Increasing nature connectedness not only improves well-being,' Richardson adds. 'It improves pro-nature attitudes and behaviours which as we are increasingly seeing is critical.'

There is a simple explanation behind the difference between noting three good things about your life and choosing to look for three good things in nature. Nature is often totally indifferent to us. Even when we are gardening, we know that the plant does most of its growing without us coaxing it along. Focusing on the outdoors rather than ourselves not only helps rewire our brains to look for the good, it also stops us from focusing entirely on ourselves.

This made a lot of sense to me. Even on days that I didn't really want to review, I could still remember the sound of the goldfinches as they bounced through the air in the street that I was walking down or the sight of the bauble seeds of a plane tree out of my window. Even when I hadn't left the house, I could still find three good things in nature, such as the starlings squabbling over my garden bird feeders, the patterns made by sunlight filtering through leaves and the way my indoor orchid plants were slowly pushing out more flowers. Often, I wanted to find more and so was more likely to decide it was worth going outside, after all. It was a gentler way of thinking back about how I had been that day and of looking forward to more of nature's richness the next day too. Now I call this 'counting the snowdrops', to remind me that even on those greyest of days, tiny good things are visible.

I often talk about snowdrops when discussing depression with others, not least because even non-gardeners know what these flowers are and therefore indulge my ramblings a little longer. But because they flower in the gloomy months, it is also a little easier not to seem as though I am slipping into the 'Cheer up, it might never happen' trap. Mental illness won't be solved merely by looking on the bright side. But mental muscle to deal with the sicker days stops the illness getting any more of you. And that's a fight worth having, even if your chief weapon seems nothing bigger than a tiny, white winter flower.

CHAPTER FOUR

Walking the Black Dog

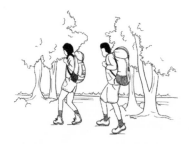

It was a miserable day when we climbed Haystacks in the Lake District. This fell was writer Alfred Wainwright's favourite: he took his last walk here and his ashes are scattered on its slope. It 'stands unabashed and unashamed in the midst of a circle of much loftier fells, like a shaggy terrier in the company of foxhounds' he wrote in his *A Pictorial Guide to the Lakeland Fells*.[1] That may be, but when my partner and I set off for the summit, our feelings were rather lower.

John has depression, which he has struggled with for much of his adult life. When his illness became particularly bad following an accident in which he suffered brain damage, he decided to speak publicly about being an MP who needed treatment. This was long before we were together – long before I even knew him – but at the time I admired him hugely for being honest when it was still rather difficult for people in public life to be so. He received a great deal of sympathy; his drawer still bulges with kind letters from other MPs who were grateful that John had decided not to hide what was keeping him away from work. *Newsnight* ran an interview with him and many journalists wrote supportive pieces. But, in private, depression doesn't feel admirable at all and, while sympathy is so helpful, it doesn't make the illness go away.

When we started our relationship, a diary piece appeared in one of the newspapers pointing out that both of us had written about our mental health problems: a rather less glamorous set of things in common than most couples would aspire to. Some people remarked that it must make it easier for both of us as we understood what the other was going through, and in many ways this was true; though our illnesses manifested themselves differently, we have shared ways of coping with one another, and when one of us is feeling strong, they can look after the other with a great deal of empathy and experience. Of course, it is far, far harder when both of us have black dogs biting at our heels at the same time. We have had some dark times as a result. In fact, the onset of my illness led to a deterioration in John's mental health as a result of the strain of being my main carer. He was referred to a psychiatrist and a psychotherapist to help him cope. Caring for someone with depression is far more difficult than just offering hugs and sympathy.

John was in a particularly low patch when we arrived at Gatesgarth for our walk in October 2017. While I would never agree with his own description of himself as a 'grumpy bugger' when he's ill, I had by this point learned that hugs and sympathy were in fact the last things he wanted, and so was keeping a quiet distance from him as we started walking. It was a damp day and the fells were rather smudgy above us. The ground was spongy with water, even as it rose up towards Scarth Gap. And as we started to ascend the steep path, John told me he didn't want to walk. He didn't feel like it. He couldn't do it. Several times, he turned back and started stomping down the path towards the car. Eventually, I persuaded him to give it another fifteen minutes, and then another. My reasoning to myself was that at the very least he wouldn't feel worse after doing the walk and seeing what waited for us at the summit.

We walked on. I left John ten metres behind me, and busied myself with inspecting the ferns and fungi growing along the path. I found my first scarlet waxcaps – near-luminous mushrooms – and several different types of moss. Behind us Buttermere yawned into its valley. We were the only walkers on the fell. All we could hear was the trudge, trudge, trudge of our own feet, the occasional sheep, and birds. I imagine the inside of John's head felt rather louder, though, even though he continued to walk in silence.

After Scarth Gap, it seemed a shame to turn back and walk down again. John agreed, so we scrambled up over the rocks and past some sheep who looked rather concerned that we were climbing the fell when a mist was looming over some of those loftier fells. Wainwright warns that 'if you attempt this walk in mist then you had better kneel down and pray for safe deliverance'. Perhaps I was wrong in presuming that the walk might make John feel a bit better.

We watched the mist and the mist watched us as we carried on. It held back, hovering over the nearby High Crag and then, just as we reached the summit, it stomped off and the sun broke out over us. The tarn at the summit was inky, but behind us Buttermere and Crummock Water were enjoying their own Turner skies. John started to talk. He didn't have much to say, still, but light was clearly breaking into his mind, too.

As we walked down past bogs where the orange seedheads of asphodel and the strappy leaves of carnivorous butterwort lingered after the summer, we even held short conversations. I showed John tiny lady's mantle plants, and noticed that he was pausing to take photos, rather than fixing his eyes firmly on his feet. We walked the last kilometre in the gloaming and drove home, happy. Wainwright's description of this walk turned out to be spot on: 'One can forget even a raging toothache on Haystacks.'

Of course, walking up Haystacks didn't cure John's depression: he had many more bad days that autumn, and in the years since. Indeed, he suspects he will have it to some degree for the rest of his life. Both of us are very active, spending our free time cycling or swimming, and exercising in the great outdoors has not stopped us from suffering. But that walk undoubtedly helped him to work through the symptoms of that illness. And while John has mild depression, walking isn't just for those whose mental health problems are at his end of the spectrum. In fact, psychiatrists believe that walking the black dog can even help patients who spend a large amount of their time in hospital.

Trees in Hospitals

Dr Jacob Krzanowski is a sustainability scholar at the Royal College of Psychiatrists and is particularly interested in how outdoor walking can help inpatients on mental health wards. He has run a walking group for inpatients with severe conditions in the grounds of the Bethlem Royal Hospital in Beckenham and was struck by the feedback from those who attended the long, slow walks in the 'gorgeous' grounds. He is now setting up walking groups in hospitals across England through the Green Walking Project.

The purpose of these groups is ultimately to get patients outdoors, active and enjoying nature. However, Dr Krzanowski also thinks something as simple as a walking group can help 'revamp the current models of how we care for people with mental illnesses'. He explains:

Walks in green spaces are interesting because their benefit appears to draw from a number of implicitly therapeutic areas including fostering relationships, supporting a sense of agency, and exposure to the natural world. Elements such as conversation, personal reflection and exploration while surrounded by natural sounds, sights and smells are all important. In that sense, they encourage us to take quite seriously the simpler and very easily disregarded aspects of mental healthcare.

Within the NHS, the relatively humble asks of our project give space for cooperation across professional bodies – including psychiatrists, occupational therapists, nurses and activity coordinators – which opens lines of communication in hospital treatment. Emphasis on green spaces in the inpatient setting also creates opportunities to bridge

the divide between inpatient and community services, by creating
the option to continue in a walking programme following a patient's
discharge.

Pressures on the wider healthcare system are such that often
improving care at the interpersonal level, and across the system,
would require a challenging and complicated intervention. The hope is
that these changes and green initiatives inspire others to speak more
openly about how we can continue to improve care for those with
mental illnesses.

Nature, on the other hand, has nothing to do with the patient.
The hospital exists to treat the person, but the trees around it are
just minding their own business and are totally uninterested. This
is handy for anyone with a mental illness, but especially so for
someone who might have spent the past five years on an inpatient
ward. Your life can feel totally defined by and centred around your
illness. Outside society can seem terrifying and judgemental. Trees,
on the other hand, don't care at all.

Approaching an old tree is like walking up to a dinosaur or a
great blue whale to say hello. These ancient pachyderms put us
in our place, viewing our lives as just a few seasons flitting past
their centuries of growth. The oldest tree in Britain is believed to
have been growing for between 2000 and 3000 years. This is the
Fortingall Yew in Perthshire. It is a twisting, warty, hunched and
craggy mammoth, so big that its trunk has split in two and local tales
include funeral processions passing through the arch in between
the two splints of its hulking body. It has seen humans struggling

and celebrating since the Bronze Age. And it has remained entirely indifferent to all of them.

Even resting your hand against the trunk of one of these trees feels as though you are giving over your cares to a great old friend, one you can lean on without fear of being let down. Inside that bulk, the tree is noisy with sap moving through it like blood through our veins. But on the outside it is silent, not popping up with platitudes about how what doesn't kill you makes you stronger, or how a positive attitude is all you need to feel better. Trees silently support one another, forming underground networks of mycorrhizal fungi which can pass food and signals between one another. Some trees can be quietly sick but be fed and nursed entirely by those around them. They can also warn others nearby of attacks, releasing pheromones when an animal decides to start munching on their leaves. The other trees release a bitter-tasting chemical into their leaves and the diner is deterred.

I have never really understood why so many people agree with Keats' description of autumn as a 'season of mists and mellow fruitfulness'.[2] Oh, there are mists, hanging over rivers where the water is warmer than the air. But there is nothing mellow about autumn. It is far more colourful and sensuous than any other season. The falling leaves create a spicy scent in the air. Cherry trees look as though they are fishing rods with their bright catches arranged along them. Bryony berries in the hedges, crab apples heavy with fruit and the plop-plop-plop of conkers and acorns falling from the trees are not watercolour, mellow sights and sounds, but nature's fireworks at the end of the growing season. Walking in a woodland at this time of year is one of the greatest pleasures of being alive.

But whenever you encounter trees, they have something to offer. In the winter, a tree looks more complicated from a distance, its bare twigs scratching the sky. Some of those branches have dramatic form, as on the oak. Other trees reveal their grace at this time of the year: the hornbeam, for instance, has a growth habit so neat that you might wonder whether someone secretly gives it a haircut from time to time. Poplars form long stripes on the horizon. Willows are red- or golden-stemmed against grey and brown fields. Birches are a deep purple.

When you get to know a tree in winter, you wonder why people get so upset that the leaves have fallen. Wintry trees have so much intricacy to explore. Their bark, for instance, is fascinating, and you notice it more at this time of the year. There's the London plane, which is famous for having bark that sheds like skin and is therefore handy in a city where pollution clings to everything. But less well-recognised is how beautiful that bark is. It's a coat of many colours; splodges and blodges of creams, greens, yellows, browns and reds. The sweet chestnut, *Castanea sativa*, which grows wild across Europe and parts of Asia, has prickly cases and edible fruits, but have you spotted how its bark is a cable-knit of lines and triangles?

The lichens, fungi and mosses living on a tree's lower slopes stand out rather more in the winter, too. Some of these tiny hangers-on are stunningly beautiful. There are shaggy lichens which look like grey tufts of hair hanging from an ageing tree and bright yellow blodgy lichens like *Xanthoria parietina*. In the leaf litter below beech trees grows my favourite fungus, the green elfcup, *Chlorociboria aeruginascens*. This has impossibly bright green-blue fruiting bodies. Fungus has a vegetative part which grows in its host called the mycelium. Green elfcup mycelium is bright blue, and stains any wood that it grows on that colour. The first time I found this mycelium under trees in Richmond Park, I thought it had come from a painted fence post. But it was, in fact, painted entirely by nature. It is rare to find the fruiting bodies of the green elfcup, but it is rarer still to fail to find at least one thing about a great tree that doesn't inspire you to wonder at the magnificence and intricacy of nature.

The first blossom comes in the deep midwinter, on the bare branches of the early-flowering cherries such as *Prunus x subhirtella*. These aren't native to Britain, but they are often planted along streets and in parks, yet few people realise that they are supposed to flower from November through to early February. More often, their dainty pale pink flowers are assumed to be a harbinger of climate change, or at the very least of an unusually sheltered spot.

As the days warm a little, the sap starts to wake in a deciduous tree. On sunny days, you can see the change that nature's alarm clock brings about in these great beasts. Rest your hand against the trunk of a tree in warm sunlight and the bark feels warm and dry, like the hands of an elderly woman. The buds on a horse chestnut stay fat and shiny through the winter, like clusters of beetles, before swelling as the leaves clamour to stream out. Branches gain a fuzziness of new growth. The tree hosts parties of birds that are hunting for nest material, building nests and shouting beautifully at one another. Some birds nest in the trees themselves: if you're ever in a woodland and hear a creaking sound like someone stepping on an old floorboard, look up into the branches for a great spotted woodpecker. Their pecks are so fast that they sound less like tapping and more like something large groaning. They burrow into the wood of an old or damaged tree to make their nests and to extract food. The adults have black-and-white spotted bodies and bright red bottoms, while their children have bright red heads. They do not hide quite as well as their relatives the green woodpeckers, which often explore on the ground, flying away like little Spitfires from startled walkers.

In January, the real wild blossom appears on the wild plum, *Prunus domestica*, followed by the sloe, *Prunus spinosa*. Both have white flowers. Then the colour joins them on wild apples and cultivated cherry trees. Magnolias open their waxy blooms, which evolved to be so thickset because they turned up before the bees and are instead pollinated by beetles, which are less dainty with their feet. Of course, in spring, our eyes are often drawn to the base of the trees, where bluebells, wild garlic and anemones bloom under the fresh green canopy.

New leaves are freshly-laundered, but they fade to a richer green over the weeks that follow. A summer tree is the one children draw: a fat lollipop trunk with a fluffy green blob on top. Lingering in the dense shade of an oak tree or the golden dappled light underneath beeches slows all of us down a little. One evening when my mental health was very poor and I was once again off work, I saw a small parcel of a bird perched on the lower branches of an oak. I lifted my binoculars and was greeted by a pair of indignant amber eyes: it was a little owl, hiding in the dusky shade.

Forest Bathing

It turns out that walking in a woodland at any time of year is more than just a pleasure, though. Trees are particularly handy when it comes to dealing with mental illness. Western medicine has recently started to take an interest in a traditional Japanese practice called 'forest bathing', whereby people walk incredibly slowly through a woodland for two hours, taking in their surroundings. Frankly, when I first heard about this, I thought it sounded like total mumbo jumbo and the sort of thing enjoyed by people who hang wind chimes in their gardens and play *Spirit of the Panpipes* CDs while drinking particularly disgusting herbal tea. But, as with the mindfulness practices that we encountered in the previous chapter, 'forest bathing' does have quite a lot of decent research backing it up as a means of managing mental illness.

Dr Qing Li is a medic at the Nippon Medical School in Tokyo and a visiting fellow at Stanford University. He enjoys forest bathing himself, but has also conducted a number of experiments to work out whether it really does improve mental health and, if so, why. His work has found that forest bathing lowers the stress hormones cortisol and adrenaline, suppresses the 'fight or flight' system, lowers blood pressure, boosts the immune system and improves sleep quality.

There's research showing that the colours of nature, especially green, are particularly good for our minds, and that the 'fractal patterns' made by plants and trees have a similar calming effect. This taps into the theory of 'biophilia', which is that we have an evolutionary need to connect with nature. Li isn't just interested in what we can see when we are in a forest, but also in our other senses, and particularly what we can smell.

Forest air, he writes in his book *Shinrin-Yoku: The Healing Art of Forest Bathing*, is full of something called phytoncides, which are a tree's natural oils to help it defend itself. Evergreen trees have much higher stores of these oils, which is why pine forests, for instance, smell so much stronger than deciduous ones. Li ran an experiment with twelve healthy middle-aged men who spent three nights sleeping in hotel rooms into which he diffused essential tree oil. They went about their days as usual, though with limited amounts of exercise. The results found that exposure to the phytoncides increased the number of a type of white blood cell known as natural killer cells, which can prevent cancer and kill cells that have been infected with viruses. The men had lower levels of stress hormones, slept longer and reported lower scores for tension, anxiety, anger, fatigue and confusion.[3]

Li also reports another study from Japan which found that the smell of one phytoncide called D-limonene was 'more effective than antidepressants for lifting mood and ensuring emotional wellbeing in patients with mental health disorders'.[4] This means that as well as recommending a two-hour walk in a forest once a month, he also thinks people should diffuse essential oils of phytoncides in their homes and workplaces to maintain their well-being. These are pretty big claims, and it's worth pointing out that this study, which took place in 1995, once again only involved twelve people who were given citrus fragrances to smell. It claims that the results of this very small study 'indicated that the doses of antidepressants necessary for the treatment of depression could be markedly reduced' and that 'the treatment with citrus fragrance normalised neuroendocrine hormone levels and immune function and was rather more effective than antidepressants'.[5]

The limited research sounded interesting enough. But even though I love walking, I was still uncomfortable about doing something called 'forest bathing'. My apprehension grew still further when I read Li's suggestion that this two-hour walk should cover merely five kilometres, and that I should turn off all technology and be totally alone in my senses while doing it. Not only was I being encouraged to be the sort of person who wafted essential oils around them, I was also being forced to disconnect from the rest of the world for what felt – at least to a busy and rather adrenaline-addicted political journalist – like a very long time.

Li is clear that forest bathing isn't just going for a normal walk. He instructs forest bathers to walk 'aimlessly and slowly' and 'let nature enter through your ears, eyes, nose, mouth, hands and feet'. This includes listening out for birds and the sounds of tree foliage moving in the breeze; looking at the different shades of green and the light; smelling the fragrance of the forest; tasting 'the freshness of the air as you take deep breaths'; and touching a tree.[6]

As a result of this work, Japan now has certified forest-bathing sites, which need to meet a number of criteria including having more than two 'forest-therapy roads' which are at least five kilometres in length, with wide paths, gentle slopes, water, a variety of plants and not too dark a canopy. Finnish researchers were intrigued by whether they could replicate this in their own highly-forested country and used government funding to set up nature trails, which were so successful they've been replicated across northern Europe. In her book, *The Nature Fix: Why Nature Makes Us Happier, Healthier, and More Creative*, journalist Florence Williams reports that the researchers 'surveyed the hikers who use them, and found that 79 per cent said their moods had improved, with greater boosts in those who walked the longer loop (6.6 kilometres) than the shorter loop (4.4 kilometres)'.[7]

We don't have the same formal network of forest-therapy centres in the UK, but there is nonetheless a network of sites in England and Scotland that meet these criteria very easily: Forestry Commission land (in Wales this is now managed by Natural Resources Wales and in Northern Ireland the Forest Service). The Forestry Commission is the government department responsible for managing woodlands and encouraging public enjoyment of many of those sites. Its paths tend to be well-maintained, wide, long and with fascinating diversity on the surrounding forest floor. Which is presumably why the Forestry Commission now runs formal forest-bathing sessions. In Scotland, the Commission set up a programme called 'Branching Out', which worked with the local NHS services to give people being treated for serious mental health problems three hours of woodland activities every week for three months. This wasn't just forest bathing, or health walks, as the activity was known, presumably to reassure any Scots worried that they might be being asked to do something a bit 'hippy'; it also included conservation activities, bushcraft and environmental art such as willow sculptures.

The project was particularly aimed at people who were less likely to be connected to nature and from deprived backgrounds, and two evaluations in 2009 and 2016 found that not only did participants report an improvement in their mental well-being, they were also less likely to drop out from the course, even though they were what healthcare professionals described as 'hard to reach' (i.e. the sort of person who would run a mile from a therapy room). The 2016 evaluation found that 'improvements in mental health and vitality as a result of the scheme are particularly marked for participants with more severe mental health problems before they entered the programme'. It also saved money: perhaps as much as £13,000 per patient.[8]

Doctors in Ireland were so impressed by the Branching Out programme that they set up their own programme called 'Woodlands For Health'. Patients were prescribed a space on the course of forest activities, and an evaluation of the project in 2014 found that participants' mood improved by 75 per cent, their sleep by 66 per cent and their thoughts of suicide declined by 82 per cent.[9]

That forests are being used to treat people with severe mental health problems who don't normally access nature gives the lie to the claim so often made by class warriors that the Natural Health Service is all very well and good if you're posh. Of course, there are satellite industries springing up in the UK offering 'forest bathing' at an amusingly high price: one expensive hotel near me in Cumbria offers a luxury spa and forest-bathing minibreak. But while people will always try to cash in on anything that has demand attached to it, the core activity remains as near to free as possible, and open to all. Yet it is worth remembering that in February 2010, a report commissioned by the government into health inequalities found that people who benefit the most from contact with nature are those from deprived backgrounds.[10]

Yes, you need a suitable pair of shoes and a good coat, but these items can be borrowed, bought very cheaply from a charity shop or given to you by a friend. If you have a friend who is struggling with their mental health but really has no money at all to buy the basic items they need to go for a forest walk, then the best present you could ever give them is a pair of cheap trainers. If you are a GP or mental health support worker, you might want to refer your patient on to a local charity that runs a clothing bank so that they can pick up a free pair of shoes. These obstacles are not insurmountable.

Many organisations, including the Forestry Commission, are also becoming increasingly aware of the need to improve access for disabled people to their sites. Wider, level paths mean your wheelchair can take you through the forest. Some nature reserves offer mobility scooter hire. People who haven't been physically active for a long time or who have suffered a physical illness, such as a heart problem, can also ease into walking. You can start slowly, walk a short distance, and incorporate it into your daily routine. One woman I met with a mental illness ditched her commute across London and walked into work every day: it took her an extra half an hour, but it kept her sane. And it saved on the Tube fare.

The Queen's Wood

I thought I was already quite good at connecting with nature in a woodland. For a couple of years now, I've tried to lean my hand against one tree every day, admiring the patterns and scars of its trunk, and peering up into its canopy. With the oldest of trees, it felt as though I was paying homage to a great being, and I found myself moved by the indifference of the ancient plant above me. Nevertheless, moving slowly, not taking photos and obeying instructions like 'drink in the flavour of the forest and release your sense of joy and calm'?[11] This felt uncomfortable and cheesy. Still, it couldn't make things worse, could it? So I decided to try, and made my way to a forest-bathing session in the UK.

The Queen's Wood in Highgate, north London, is next to a thrumming, busy road. The wood itself is thrumming too, with birdsong, walkers and a group of children from the local forest school nursery, who are all stuffed into their winter clothing like overfilled shopping bags. In one corner of the wood, Claire de Boursac is starting her weekly forest-therapy session. We are sitting in a circle in a wooden cabin, our phones off. There's a box of tissues on the floor, as you'd find in any good therapy session. Claire even uses the sort of words and phrases you might expect to hear in a counselling room: she suggests that this is a time for us to connect with ourselves and explains that, during the session, she will help us experience nature better. We take some deep breaths and sniff at a bottle of hinoki oil (an extract from the hinoki cypress tree), before leaving the cabin behind.

No one in our group talks during the session. Much of it is spent in total silence, punctuated only by Claire suggesting certain activities – what she calls 'invitations'. We don't really interact much as we meander ever so slowly through the wood. There's a nice tarmac path which must be very handy if you're pushing a buggy or in a wheelchair, but we don't stick to it, making our own way between the oaks, hornbeams and beeches. This is not really a walk. We don't travel very far at all, and the pace is so slow that at times we're almost moving backwards. Only at the very end do we sit together on a fallen tree, drinking nettle and mint tea, discussing some of the things that struck us over the past two hours.

This session made me realise how many of my senses I put on standby. Claire worked hard to help me switch them back on, running through gentle exercises that took in each sense. First, we picked herbs from the community garden beds, smelling the lavender leaves and tasting the young lemon balm. Then, we learned to switch our focus from near to far. The trees around me came into sharper detail: I noticed the vivid green notches on the bark of a young holly and the shining streaks of rain on a hornbeam trunk. Even looking up through the twigs at the top of the canopy made me realise how casual my glances normally are: I noticed the spaces in between different trees' crowns and the swelling buds on the hornbeams.

We touched the things around us, picking up leaf mould, placing the backs of our hands against moss on tree trunks, seeing how it felt when pressing our cheeks against the bark. Spotting a very knobbly mossy stump, I took my shoes and socks off, and stood on it. The wood was damp and cool. It pressed against the arches of my feet, which I suddenly realised felt tired and stiff after months of marathon training. Later, I found huge hummocks of frogspawn in a pond, and pushed my fingers into the gelatinous mass. I started to notice smaller sensations, like the cool, damp air on my cheek and the leaves under my shoes as I walked.

We were walking on a morning in early March, just after a rain shower. The moisture made it easier to smell the wood, giving us a glimpse of what it must be to be a dog that is constantly distracted by its nose. We focused on the forest's soundscape too: great tits, song thrushes, blue tits and long-tailed tits were all busy setting out their territories. A great spotted woodpecker was making his creaking and groaning sounds as he set to work on a tree trunk above us. But again, when we really tried to listen, other sounds became louder. Water was dropping from one leaf to another and then flopping on to the woodland floor. A branch creaked. A twig fell.

Walking without any purpose meant we found ourselves being drawn to certain things. I found a hornbeam which was clearly struggling to make its way in the shade of a mature oak. Its thin trunk zig-zagged towards the light, creating elbows and knock knees as it went. I was attracted to its shape, and spent a few minutes feeling my way along the smooth bark. The tree felt wobbly, unstable. I spent a while thinking about a passage from Peter Wohlleben's *The Hidden Life of Trees*, which describes how young trees wait in the shadow of forest giants for their moment to mature:

> You can observe for yourself whether young trees are playing the waiting game or putting on a growth spurt. Take a look at the branches of a small silver fir or beech. If the tree is obviously wider than it is tall, then the young tree is in waiting mode. The light it is getting is not sufficient to create the energy it needs to grow a taller trunk, and therefore, the youngster is trying to catch the few leftover rays of sunlight as efficiently as possible. To do this, it lengthens its branches out sideways and grows special ultra-sensitive leaves or needles that are adapted to shade. Often you can't even make out the main shoot on trees like these; they resemble flat-topped bonsai. One day, it's finally time. The mother tree reaches the end of her life or becomes ill. The showdown might take place during a summer storm. As torrents of rain pour down, the brittle trunk can no longer support the weight

of several tons of crown, and it shatters. As the tree hits the ground, it snaps a couple of waiting seedlings. The gap that has opened up in the canopy gives the remaining members of the kindergarten the green light, and they can begin photosynthesizing to their hearts' content. Now their metabolism gets into gear, and the trees grow sturdier leaves and needles that can withstand and metabolize bright light. This stage lasts between one and three years. Once it is over, it's time to get a move on. All the youngsters want to grow now, and only those that go for it and grow straight as an arrow toward the sky are still in the race.[12]

This hornbeam was waiting, I told myself, but looking up at the oak that it had grown close to, I wasn't sure it was going to get its moment for a long while yet. The big tree was straight, healthy and not showing the stout girth and dead wood of an elderly giant. I looked around at the other saplings, wondering which one might win the race, and noticed that the neighbouring hornbeam had green buds all over its twigs. Turning back to my tree, I couldn't spot a single emerging leaf. I reached up and snapped a twig. It was dead.

I was rather annoyed by this. Claire had asked us to turn to a tree we felt especially drawn to and think about why we might want to spend time with it. I had been telling myself some rather contrived story about how long it takes to heal and grow, and how the scars we gathered along the way could still be beautiful, like the zig-zagging trunk of this young tree. And in fact, it wasn't a young tree, it was a dead tree. Serves me right for being so dreadfully whimsical.

Wohlleben describes what happened to my hornbeam in his very next sentences:

The cards are stacked against those free spirits who think they can meander right or left as the mood takes them and dawdle before they stretch upward. Overtaken by their comrades, they find themselves in the shadows once again. The difference is that it is even darker under the leaves of their cohort that has pulled ahead than it was under their mothers. The teenagers use up the greater part of what weak light remains; the stragglers give up the ghost.

It was then that the beautifully awful nature of forest life struck me. Woodlands seem so tranquil, so balanced, but they are brutal places. My tree had spent decades waiting for its moment, but had never made it. Instead, as I looked closer, I saw the orange spots of fungi starting to take over the bark, and the wood itself was soft when I pressed my fingernail into it. This tree was serving its purpose in another way. Soon it would end up feeding not just the mighty oak it had seeded itself so close to, but also the thrumming wildlife of this woodland.

There seemed to be no neat life lesson here, nothing you'd want to write on a fridge magnet or share on social media. I'd come here hoping to connect with myself, and instead I'd been drawn to a tree that was secretly dead. After nearly three years of counselling, CBT and schema therapy, I was pretty adept at thinking deeply about why I felt the way I did about something, yet this tree had confounded me.

On the cycle home, my mind ran up and down the dead trunk of that tree. I wondered why I was so annoyed by it. It seemed an inconvenient intrusion into what had largely been a celebration of the beauty of woodlands, not the sadness. After about six miles of pedalling past hair salons, upmarket bakeries and neon-lit nail spas, I started to conclude that I was annoyed by how messy and unfair life is, even my lovely, fortunate life. I had so much to be thankful for, but I had spent the past few months deeply annoyed that my illness meant I was still missing out on opportunities at work. Others were, like the saplings around my dead hornbeam, pulling ahead with so much proud vigour, while I had to take yet more days off to rest my exhausted mind. I was angry with the people who I suspected looked down on me for my continuing weakness, and envious of those whose lives seemed easier.

I won't torture the metaphor further, as I was obviously not dead. I was still on my bike, in fact, pedalling towards my study so I could carry on writing this book. Things were looking considerably better for me than they were for that tree back in the Queen's Wood. This wasn't a divine message from the wood; it was merely an opportunity for me to understand why I felt the way I did about certain things I'd seen there. It was CBT without any walls and with no tissue box in sight.

I found thinking about all this rather helpful, as my resentment at the setbacks caused by being ill had been humming in the distance of my mind, like the road at the edge of the wood. It wasn't something I'd really taken the time to think through properly. Now, a dead tree had forced me to. Reflecting further, I realised that I had been useful in other ways while ill: writing about having PTSD seemed to help other people with the illness, and make mental health problems seem just a little less secret. It wasn't as big a loss as I often told myself it was.

Perhaps it was the way in which we had gradually switched on all our senses or perhaps it was taking an extended period of time to enjoy the wood without distraction. But at the end of the session, I felt calmer and more alert than I had done for days. I wrote 4000 words afterwards, which suggested that I hadn't wasted my time by taking two hours away from my desk.

The Tyranny of Phones

One of the things I found hardest about the prospect of the forest-bathing session was the idea that I would have to turn my phone off for two hours to do it. In fact, I am not sure it has *ever* been off for that long. I have all the excuses lined up: I'm a political journalist in a world where news feels old ten minutes after it has broken. It often breaks at inconvenient times of the day. I've filed stories from children's birthday parties, crammed Tube carriages, pub toilets and, of course, my bed. You need your phone to stay afloat across the raging storms of British politics. Even when I'm not filing a story, my notifications are buzzing constantly with MPs getting in touch to discuss something that they're up to or wanting an idle gossip. Some also get in touch at inconvenient times of the day; there's one who thinks it is a good idea to send me interesting news stories that he's just seen (and that I've already read) at 11 p.m. on a Friday, for instance. But do I really need to pick my phone up hundreds of times a day? How often am I doing so because something has actually happened, and how often because I feel the need to check my screen more anxiously than an intensive care nurse checks on their patients?

I'm not the only person who finds their wrist twitching to pick up my phone throughout the day. A report by UK communications regulator Ofcom in 2018 discovered that people now check their smartphones every twelve minutes of the day when they are awake. For two in five adults, this starts within five minutes of first waking, and 37 per cent of adults are still checking their phones in bed, five minutes before they turn their lights off for the night.[13]

The report found much that was positive about what it called the 'decade of digital dependency'. Phones and the Internet allow people to work more flexibly and stay in touch with friends and family. But then again, 15 per cent of people said being online all the time made them feel as though they were constantly at work, and 54 per cent admitted that their devices interrupt face-to-face conversations with friends and family. And 43 per cent of adults felt they were spending too much time online.

Smartphone addiction is an unresolved battleground in mental health. Many argue that it is the key driver behind the explosion in diagnosed mental illnesses among children and teenagers. Others say this is just the latest moral panic: people fretted about the impact of the novel when it first appeared, and now we're worrying about something that, by and large, makes life much easier. There's even a debate about whether phones are addictive in and of themselves. Why are they any different to books that you 'just can't put down', for instance?

For many people with mental illnesses, their phone means they can find other people who are suffering from the same conditions. It means their friends can check up on them regularly. But, of course, there is a dark side. Social media giants are increasingly being held responsible for tragedies involving young people dying by suicide having spent many hours browsing graphic content about self-harm and suicide on their phones, or who have been the victims of prolonged and vicious cyberbullying. Being a teenager is hideous enough without the crushing pressure to have the right number of followers on Instagram and to present a perfect, airbrushed life to your peers. Teenagers use digital retouching apps which make their faces appear almost identical to one another, desperately removing what they see as being blemishes but which are in reality part of their true identities, often beautifully so. The sense of self that develops as a result of a life online is rarely a strong one; a skin as easy to break as the surface of water.

Professor Miles Richardson, whose work on nature connectedness we encountered in the previous chapter, has also studied the link between phones and mental health. What he has found so far is a stunning testament to the power of nature, even when pitted against modern technology. Smartphone use can turn into a behavioural addiction, and Richardson's team examined the correlation between smartphone use and so-called nature connectedness in a group of 244 people with an average age of thirty. They found that those who were the most connected to nature spent half as much time on their phones as those who were the least. These most connected people took 90 per cent fewer selfies – around one a week instead of ten – and were 'significantly more agreeable, conscientious and open to new experiences'. The less connected people were, the more anxious they were.[14]

But, conversely, smartphones can also be a useful way of connecting with nature. Richardson also ran an app which asked people in Derby to log places where they came into contact with nature. He found 'clinically significant health improvements in mental health' in those who used the app.

Child and adolescent psychiatrists are worried that overuse of social media makes children more vulnerable to anxiety and depression, as well as cyberbullying. Jon Goldin, vice chair of the Child and Adolescent Faculty at the Royal College of Psychiatrists, warned in 2018 that parents shouldn't be giving phones to their children before they reach secondary school age.[15] Research published that year in the journal *Psychological Medicine* claimed that there was a link between soaring mental illness among children and the introduction of the Internet into young people's lives. Between 1995 and 2014, the number of people aged between four and twenty-four who reported a 'long-standing mental health condition' increased six-fold.[16] The study's lead researcher, Dr Dougal Hargreaves of Imperial College London, said the rise could be partly down to greater awareness of mental illness, but that a generation brought up on the Internet was also struggling with its ill effects:

> While some of it could be explained by better awareness and a reduction in stigma around mental health, other things such as social media and cyberbullying may well have contributed to the rise in mental health problems among young people. We know that young people say social media has a negative impact on their self-esteem, with almost half of young girls highlighting this in a recent survey.

There are also theories that smartphone use actually changes the wiring of our brains, and not for the better. In 2017, neuroradiologists examined the brains of nineteen teenagers who had been diagnosed with Internet or smartphone addictions, and a control group of nineteen similar adolescents who had no diagnosis. They found differences in the neurotransmitters which are understood to be markers for addictions, though it's not clear whether the phone rewired the brain or the brains were particularly susceptible to getting hooked on the phone.[17] The social media giants know this, too, programming the same feedback loops into their software that you find in arcade machines and, er, cocaine. This is a cycle mediated by dopamine, the reward chemical that our brains release when something good happens, like eating delicious food, having great sex, or successful social interactions. That last one happens a lot on social media. Someone likes or favourites one of your photos: dopamine hit. A notification buzzes on your phone: dopamine hit.

Where this really goes awry, though, is that we don't always get a hit with every post we create. And when the rewards are randomised, then we're in a similar world to that of the problem gambler, who keeps going because they don't quite know when they are going to get lucky. So we post more updates, hoping that this latest photo will get the requisite number of likes to make us feel rewarded. And because there isn't much effort involved in looking at our phone to check whether we've struck lucky this time, we keep looking, just in case.

Continuing to look all the way to bedtime can render us sleepless addicts. The light from our screens, much stronger and with more blue in it than the light bulbs in our homes, tricks our brain into thinking that it's still the time of day to stay awake, and suppresses the production of melatonin, the hormone that helps us sleep. We also stay awake in bed longer, staring at our phones, which means we are automatically reducing the amount of time in which our bodies can try to sleep. One American study which looked at 653 people found that the longer someone spent on their phone, the worse their sleep quality and the shorter their overall sleep time. The closer to bed a person used their smartphone, the more likely they were to have poor-quality sleep.[18]

Everyone knows what sleep deprivation does to them, even when they are healthy. But if you have a mental health problem, losing sleep can make your symptoms considerably worse. For those with psychotic illnesses or bipolar disorder, sleep deprivation can actually trigger manic episodes, psychosis or paranoia. Conversely, many people with these conditions report that taking time off to sleep for longer periods of time can actually halt the onset of these acute episodes. I have found that one of the ways of stopping a descent into paranoia is to take a day off work and sleep, often for an extra eight hours. It's not especially convenient, but then neither is vocally accusing your colleagues of plotting against you. I know which one I'd rather take.

Phone manufacturers such as Apple have recently caught up with popular concerns about screen time. You can now ask your phone to tell you how much time you are spending looking at it, how many times you pick it up and which apps you spend the most time browsing. Of course, the inherent problem with this is that you need to pick up your phone in order to find out quite how addicted you are to it, thus inviting yet another wave of notifications. You can also set your phone so that the light changes from that harsh, melatonin-suppressing blue to a mellower yellow, so your body is receiving fewer signals that it should stay awake.

But surely a better way to break smartphone addiction, or whatever name you want to give to the problems that inappropriate use of a phone can cause, is to spend less time on your phone. Being forced to switch it off for a few hours might be hideous, but then again, doing this in an outdoor setting where you suddenly become aware of what's around you could be far more pleasant than you'd imagined.

This is why some therapists choose to treat their clients not in a bare counselling room with a box of tissues, but outside, using the wonder of nature to help people relax and then talk about their problems. Walking with your therapist rather than sitting in a room feels less formal and intimidating, just as going for a walk with a friend and setting the world to rights feels perfectly natural. But it's not just that you've left the therapy room behind; you're also experiencing the benefits of being outside. Natural views help calm people, and help them recover better from physical and mental problems. To be opening up about painful experiences while using the anaesthetic of nature might mean that the therapy sessions themselves become a little more bearable. Even the costs of getting outdoors are tiny sums compared to the amount of money a person could save themselves in extra prescriptions, loss of earnings and perhaps even spending on things that temporarily relieve the pain, but really cause a longer-term deterioration in health, such as alcohol.

The Black Dog Walks

Jake Tyler knows all about how easy it is to spend money on things that numb your mental pain for a day but make it worse for weeks.

He had always felt depressed. He just didn't realise that 'being a grumpy bastard' wasn't an aspect of his character but an illness. In fact, he didn't realise this until he had been alive for thirty years.

How do people with serious mental illness cope for this long before a diagnosis? Well, the answer is that they still use medication, just not the sort available on the NHS. Jake self-medicated with drink and illegal drugs, both of which were readily available given he worked in the hospitality sector. Self-medication sounds deliberate, but most of the time it is an unconscious attempt to numb the pain of mental illness. Self-harm also falls into this category, and indeed heavy drinking and drugs are a form of self-harm, of regulating mental pain by causing physical pain. This is why it is strange that Western culture trivialises alcoholism. It isn't any funnier than the mental illness that drives it.

Naturally, self-medication doesn't actually work. And so, eventually, Jake fell apart. When he ended up in his GP's surgery, hearing the words 'depression', he felt a massive relief, he tells me, as we troop past the very first flowers of spring at Kew Gardens. 'I realised that this wasn't me: it wasn't my fault,' he explains. This is so important. A diagnosis often means a great deal to people with physical or mental problems, partly because it's the start of them being able to understand what is going on, and partly because of the relief derived from knowing they are not to blame.

Stuck at home and too sick to work, Jake found his mother – a mental health nurse – nagging him to get out of bed and outside. He had resisted a prescription for antidepressants because he wondered whether 'I might be able to get my shit together on my own'. As part of this, he decided to take his mother's dog for regular walks.

And unlike the times in bed when it was just Jake and his thoughts shouting in his ears, he found that this didn't make things worse. In fact, Jake became so reliant on walking that one day when he and the dog got home, the creature fell asleep almost instantly. Jake realised that he had managed to walk fifteen miles without even realising.

Why had he become so hooked on walking? Jake says it gave him a chance to think through his problems without drowning in them. Given one of his coping mechanisms had been largely to drown his sorrows in alcohol, Jake did need to confront them. Walking helped him do just that without making him want to run a mile. 'It made me feel more human,' he explains. It's difficult to describe how effective mental illness is at making you feel less human. It numbs you, and often makes you feel as though you are just existing, rather than living. Bringing alive his senses on a walk outdoors helped Jake fight that numb feeling.

In fact, he loved feeling more human so much that when a rather bizarre idea popped into his head, Jake didn't dismiss it, but instead decided to take it up, embarking on a walk that would take him two years. 'When I had this idea to walk around the UK raising awareness and money for mental health, it felt like an epiphany,' he says, still sounding excited, even though he is just days from finishing that 3000-mile walk. 'It just meant I had a purpose, that there was something I could actually do.' He set to work, plotting where he would walk, and how he would manage to get enough money in order to survive while he did it.

There was one problem, though: for Jake to raise enough money to be able to make this trek, he needed to ask his friends for help. And none of his friends even knew that Jake was mentally ill. It took what Jake calls 'a big leap of courage' to set up a fundraising page in which he explained what was going on. He had no idea how his friends would respond. As is the case for so many people today, Jake was surprised when they all rushed back to him, not just with sympathy but also stories of their own mental problems.

As his project, which he dubbed 'The Black Dog Walks', got underway, Jake realised that he really had no idea what he was doing. Not just in the wider sense of why he should walk all the way around the country, but also in terms of what he actually needed. His shoes rubbed him so hard in the first few days of walking that he developed painful blisters. He often didn't know where he was staying or how long it would take him to get to the next spot. One night, later on in his walk, he found himself in the Cairngorms with the light fading fast and no hope of reaching his destination. On so many of these occasions, Jake ended up being saved by the kindness of strangers: an army veteran who took him home to give him talcum powder to stop the blisters, people who'd heard about his walk and offered to put him up, and a group of walkers who had found a bothy in the Cairngorms and started a fire so that the hut was marvellously warm when Jake arrived. Far from being the stereotype of a depressive – a lonely figure on a path – Jake was coming into contact with the best of humanity as he walked.

When he finished in Brighton in the autumn of 2017, Jake had no idea what he would do next. He had spent two years knowing that the next day would involve walking, and now there was nothing. But he was still upbeat because his walk had given him a long-term purpose. He knew that he wanted to work in the realm of exercise and mental health. He knew he wanted to help other people. Within a few months, a local radio station had offered him a show interviewing people with mental illnesses about their own experiences. He hadn't really set off with a destination in mind, but when the walk was over, Jake found his life made a bit more sense. He still struggles with his mental health. But he now knows what to do when he's unwell. It's just that his walks are rather shorter these days.

Jake is now part of an exciting and excited group of bright young things who have made mental health their livelihoods. He's friends with Bryony Gordon, the *Telegraph* journalist whose writing about her obsessive-compulsive disorder, bulimia and battle with addiction has changed the way the media approaches mental illness. Bryony is also a firm believer in the restorative power of walking for good mental health.

Bryony was sick, and had grown sicker while writing her memoir of her illness. Feeling alone and in what she describes as a 'terrible funk', she decided that she – and others – might benefit from a walk with people who were also finding their fight with their minds difficult. She posted on Twitter that she was setting up a regular walk for people with mental health issues, and that the first one would be on Valentine's Day in Hyde Park.

Travelling to the Lido Cafe in Hyde Park, Bryony had no idea what she was setting up. She worried that no one would be there. Instead, from the twenty people who arrived on that wet Sunday morning, she has established a whole organisation dedicated to the process. Mental Health Mates, as it is called, now walks not just all around the United Kingdom, but overseas as well.

Niamh Burns set up the Edinburgh branch of Mental Health Mates. She's a press officer in her thirties who suffers with severe anxiety and depression, and she realised in 2018 that not everyone had the kind of supportive network that she relied on to get her through the hardest times. 'Setting up a group has allowed myself and others who've come along to connect with people and talk in a space without fear or judgement about our feelings and experiences,' she says. The first walk started at the Royal Botanic Garden in Edinburgh, a place I've often trudged around when trying to deal with a low patch. Niamh explains:

A walk in the fresh air for an hour or so each month gives people the opportunity to talk to one another and realise that mental health issues are just as important as physical ones. For a number of people who've come along to the walks, it's been about overcoming a shyness and nervousness in opening up about our own experiences. There's still a lot of stigma around mental health and, in my experience, families and friends who've not experienced it can find it difficult to understand. Having a walk once a month has connected me to people I would never have met and also given me a wider understanding of just how many people are looking for that connection or peer support.

Not everyone is looking for a specifically mental-health-themed walk, though. Nor does everyone have a diagnosable mental illness. But everyone does have mental health, and, just like physical health, it fares better when you put some time into looking after it. That's why Michael Di Paola set up an organisation called Freshwalks, which now runs in both Manchester and Liverpool. These guided walks on Fridays and over weekends are aimed at busy professionals who want to do a bit of networking while enjoying the great outdoors. Solicitors, accountants and others with very long working weeks and endlessly busy email inboxes turn up, pay £15, and follow Michael around the Peak District:

> It attracts really nice people. They look out for each other… the community and the sense of belonging is one massive thing I've seen. For a lot of my attendees, they're co-working or working from home and they don't get that office environment where they are surrounded by teams of people. They see the walks as a community for them.

Michael is adamant that his walks aren't a therapy group. But he thinks that everyone needs that time off to recharge their minds and work through their problems. He notices that a number of his fellow walkers particularly like the fact that he has organised the route and done his homework on the weather so that they don't have to worry about anything. 'One guy told me that this is the only time I can turn up and actually think. I don't want a map. I don't want to know where we are going.'

But though he doesn't want to offer therapy, the outdoors does it anyway. There are walkers who use the groups as a preventative measure to avoid burnout from busy jobs. One man manages his anxiety by coming along, and Michael tells the story of another conversation that showed him just what the walks meant to some of those turning up:

> The day I realised this was more of a powerful thing than what I'd set it up as was when a young man who'd only been along once before came again, and I'd seen some very dark stuff on his social media. I asked if he was okay, and he just opened up and shared a very recent personal tragedy. It turned out this was his first human contact outside his immediate family and he used the walks as a vehicle for his return

to work, to ease himself into returning and talking about what had happened.

So it's not just the walk itself that helps. It's the people who you walk with. It does stand to reason that walking the black dog is far less lonely when you're doing it in a pack.

—

CHAPTER FIVE

Racing Out of the Darkness

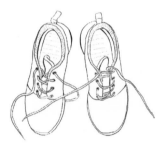

Hope Virgo must have been about fourteen when I first saw her, singing in the choir at the front of the church we both attended. She was in that peachy bloom of adolescence, dimpled cheeks and the first swelling curves of womanhood. She sang a lot in our church, her hair always immaculate and her clothes just that bit cooler than anyone else around her. Life was visibly coursing through her.

It was therefore so difficult not to notice when, a few months later, I caught sight of Hope walking down the steps of our local bookshop. She seemed bundled into a coat that was too large for her. Her cheeks were gone, her face now just two rather grey lips clamped together in a small line. I wasn't surprised when her name appeared in the list of notices of people who needed prayer: 'Hope Virgo is in hospital' it read. No one needed to ask what sort of hospital she was in: anorexia had left more than a calling card on her body.

I left the church a few months later, but over the decade that followed, I found myself wondering what had happened to Hope. I wasn't even sure if she was still alive, but I couldn't stop thinking about the way her whole body manifested the sadness in her mind. And then, one evening as I sat writing up stories from yet another political conference, an email arrived in my inbox from Hope Virgo. She was alive.

She wasn't sure if I remembered her, Hope wrote, but she was now working, smiling and campaigning for better treatment of people like her with eating disorders. She had become a keen runner who had completed a number of marathons. You may be rather surprised to learn that running might help someone who was already burning far too many calories for what they consumed. But it did and it still keeps her sane today.

It only seemed right that we discuss how this happened while out for a run. The only problem was that Hope, who was now so visibly keen to be alive, was considerably faster than me. Her 'conversational pace' turned out to be the sort of speed I saved for short bursts on the track with my running club. It's just as well, I thought, that asking questions takes up less breath.

What I learned as Hope ran and I panted alongside her was that a lot more had been going on at the church where I first saw her singing happily away. Hope had been sexually abused by someone who was supposed to be in a position of responsibility over the young people in the congregation. A hectic family life and pressure at school meant that she felt the only thing she had control over was what she ate or, increasingly, what she didn't.

In her book, *Stand Tall Little Girl*, Hope describes the efforts her family went to as they tried to coax her to eat – and how secretive she became as she either hid the food in her pockets or took herself off 'for a shower' to vomit it back up again.[1] Eventually, an ECG showed that her heart was close to stopping, and she was admitted as an inpatient to an eating disorder clinic. Her routine there was as food-obsessed as it had been at home, but here there were professionals who were entirely focused on getting Hope to eat a proper breakfast with full-fat milk – and helping her realise that she wasn't fat, but close to death.

Her nurse laid down huge pieces of poster paper in Hope's bedroom and asked her to draw the body she imagined she had. Then the nurse drew around Hope's real shape. This outline was tiny compared to the one Hope had produced. 'I stared at the paper lost for words,' she writes. 'Why couldn't I see myself as being that small? Why did I feel so huge?' Soon, she learned that anorexia, the illness that she had seen as being her friend for so long, was actually 'a manipulative, selfish bitch, and she had destroyed me'. But she was still engaged in competitive under-eating with the other girls in the hospital. They tried to hide scraps of food in their yoghurt pots, and even broke into the kitchen to throw out some bread they considered particularly calorific.

Hope was on a strict routine with even stricter rules. One of those included no exercise. In fact, patients weren't even allowed out into the grounds if they were under a certain BMI. So how did we end up running around Battersea Park together, ten years later?

It turns out that one of Hope's nurses recognised that running had been a passion long before anorexia had taken its hold. Hope longed to be able to do it again. Of course, she partly wanted to exercise so she could keep her weight down, but as we rounded another corner of the park, she explained that running for her was also about life being normal again when anorexia had made it anything but. She reached an agreement with her nurse: if she stuck to her meals and put on weight, then she could go for a short run. She now believes that this was one of the key motivations to help her recover. And in the years since, running has become a way for Hope to clear her mind of difficult thoughts.

The late afternoon sun is hanging thick through the park trees as Hope describes how a run makes her feel:

> I can work through all of my problems. And I have an order in which I do things. I tend to plan what I'm going to do when I get back, which is important to me. Then I think about stuff that's on my mind, whether it's things that I'm worried or angry about or just stuff that's happening. I definitely have bits in my runs where I run a bit harder because I'm angry with someone, but then I kind of feel like I've dealt with it. I also have all my best ideas when I'm out running. It helps me order my thoughts.

I know that I'll never be able to run a marathon in three and a half hours as Hope has done, but I also know that our minds run in the same way as we pound the pavements. I, too, find that running helps me work through problems, traumas and minor stresses in a methodical fashion that just isn't so easy when I'm stationary.

Perhaps it's the fact that I can never sink particularly deep into my thoughts when I also have to remember to breathe or when my body is whingeing that it might fancy a rest soon.

That speedy marathon that Hope ran represented another point in her recovery. She had previously trained for a marathon while restricting her calories. 'It was awful,' she says. 'I was so slow.' Of course, slow for her turns out to be the time I'm targeting for my first marathon, but nevertheless the experience made her realise that she couldn't get away with disrespecting her body if she also expected it to run fast. So, for her second marathon, she had a proper running diet, and enjoyed the process much more.

She still has to be careful, though, and has written a list of warning signs that a relapse might be on the way. The last one happened in 2016, and Hope nearly killed herself. She doesn't want to go back there, and tries to correct herself when the early warning signs start up, rather than later down the line. Those warning signs include counting calories, viewing her body in a negative way and overexercising. She explains:

> There is always a temptation for me to overexercise and start pushing myself far too hard. My friends annoy me by asking me how much longer I'm going to stay at the gym, but I know that's because they're aware that I could just stay there all morning if I don't have someone checking up on me. I run with a group of friends, too, as that helps me slow down a bit.

For a moment, I feel as though my plodding is doing Hope a service, as I have definitely slowed us down a lot.

The Running Addiction

Running for your mental health has become so common and well-understood now that it was the first thing I always mentioned when trying to explain to people what the Natural Health Service might entail. Runners would hear the words 'the great outdoors' and 'exercise' and cut me off to tell a story about how training for various long-distance feats had helped them through all manner of misery. Non-runners would nod rather wearily, trying to avoid showing their frustration that this alleged mental elixir always felt so hideous when they tried it themselves.

There are libraries of books about lives transformed by running. Bella Mackie had suffered from anxiety all her life, to the extent that she barely left the house or visited large parts of London. But when her marriage broke down, she felt a strange urge to start running. This, she explains in her book *Jog On*, led to her 'reaching parts of the city that I hadn't been able to visit in years, especially alone'. She could run where she couldn't walk:

> I could not have done this if I'd been walking – I'd tried so many times but my anxiety would break through, palms sweating and looming panic taking over. But somehow, running was different. When your brain has denied you the chance to take the mundane excursions that most people do every day, being able to pass through stalls selling 'nobody knows I'm a lesbian' T-shirts suddenly feels like a red-letter day. By concentrating on the rhythm of my feet striking the pavement, I wasn't obsessing over my breathing, or the crowds, or how far I was from home. I could be in an area my brain had previously designated

as 'unsafe' and not feel like I was going to faint. It was miraculous to me.[2]

How was this possible? Mackie had the same experience that so many runners, whether as unimpressive as me or as speedy as Hope, report. Our minds are too busy dealing with the effort of running that they simply cannot torture us in the way that they do when we are at rest. There are even books written exclusively for those who have never been sporty and who find it impossible to imagine themselves as 'runners'. Bryony Gordon has written one of them.[3] She didn't see herself as a runner, 'until, one day, I realised that I was'. Gordon now uses running to manage her obsessive-compulsive disorder. She hasn't just run the London Marathon; she's done it in her bra.

In *Outrunning the Demons*, Phil Hewitt interviews a series of people, including me, who lace up their trainers to run away from the black dog.[4] Alastair Campbell is one of his subjects. The former spin doctor to Tony Blair became addicted to the sport after going for just one run while on holiday, deciding within days to enter the London Marathon. That word 'addicted' gives the lie to one of the symptoms of Campbell's mental illness: he is a recovering alcoholic and has often mused that, with running, he has merely replaced one addiction with another.

My first run as an adult came in 2013, long before I fell ill. It didn't feel like the hit of a drug, though my friends would point out that given I've never so much as smoked tobacco, I wouldn't really know. Instead, the whole thing felt awful. My lungs screamed and my whole body felt bizarrely out of sync. I lasted ten minutes before

I stopped and walked back to my flat miserably. It was only when I joined a beginners' running club at my local gym that I discovered that the main barrier to me being able to run wasn't my lungs or the inability of my legs to know what to do. It was my mind.

The cheery running coach encouraged me to stick by him at the pace of a penguin while we ran my first ever 3k. 'I won't be able to do this,' I said, confidently. But he was so confident that I just decided to agree with him, and kept going. And I did run 3k that day. A few weeks later, I joined my local parkrun and ran 5k for the first time. I can still remember the red-faced pride that I felt, and the way the volunteers applauded me as though I'd just broken a record.

Many runners say their transition from unsporty character to someone who sees themselves as a 'runner' happened when they bought their first pair of running shoes. I had previously been trying to run in a pair of £10 trainers that I'd managed to get in the sales. They weren't particularly comfortable and, not having very much money of my own at all, I had to save for a while until I made a trip to a running shop. That visit marked the end of me considering myself too useless to run. I started to enjoy the way my mind would descend into a quiet tunnel when I ran. It would work methodically through anything I'd been worrying about, and end up happily mulling over column ideas, new arguments I was wrestling with and plans for the day. This was the 'void' that novelist Haruki Murakami says he runs to find:

> I just run. I run in a void. Or maybe I should put it the other way: I run in order to acquire a void. But, as you might expect, an occasional thought will slip into this void. People's minds can't be a complete blank. Human beings' emotions are not strong or consistent enough

to sustain a vacuum. What I mean is, the kinds of thoughts and ideas
that invade my emotions as I run remain subordinate to that void.
Lacking content, they are just random thoughts that gather around that
central void.[5]

Even long before I fell ill, I needed to acquire this void in my head.
My mind wasn't blank when I ran. It just felt as though the words
in it were being unjumbled and placed on to lined paper. Doing
a stressful job with long hours, I needed to tidy my thoughts up
reasonably regularly, and so I became a runner. I ran a half-marathon
and joined a night running group. On those trips, everything went
into a tunnel, as all you could see was the pool of light cast in
front of you by your head torch, and all you could hear was the
sound of the runner in front of you as they moved through the dark
woodlands. I ran before work, or on the way home from work, and
at the weekends. I made friends at my local parkrun, volunteering
as a marshal or scanning people's barcodes.

So when I found myself in the doctor's office, planning my
sick leave, it seemed inevitable that running would feature in my
recovery. I'd made peace with my screaming lungs by this point,
and knew that there almost always comes a point in a run when
you forget how awful you feel and start enjoying your surroundings.
But while I knew that running would help my mind, I also had to
wrestle with that mind in order to stand a chance of getting out of
the door. That's where a personal trainer came in handy. I needed
someone to force me out of the house.

Running while acutely unwell was almost as hard as it had been
when I'd just started puffing my way miserably around the block of

flats where I lived. The medication made me sluggish and I found it near-impossible to match the pace I'd comfortably reached at parkrun just a few months before. Even when I was running a series of ten-kilometre and ten-mile races for charity the following year, I had to make peace with the fact that I'd often feel as though I was running through sand. I still enjoyed the mind tunnel and I still felt much better after a run; I just wasn't running to the standard I'd come to expect of myself.

During those runs, I started to apply a mental technique that Vanda the personal trainer had taught me. If I didn't think I could manage the whole distance, it would be better to break the run down into smaller components. I could definitely manage to run to the next tree, or indeed to the end of the park. Then, once I'd got there, I could think about whether I was really able to keep going. That Socratic dialogue got me through my marathon training too – I told myself when I'd reached ten miles I could run another three miles without even thinking about it and so on. However, such mental gymnastics also helps me to manage my thoughts when my legs are still. I have learned to reason with myself when I feel so low that I am not sure whether I will survive the day. I've survived previous days without even thinking about it, I tell myself. Another one will be a piece of cake. Let's just get through this one meeting, or this one column, and see how we feel about carrying on later.

Then there's what I can see while I'm running. Counting the number of foxglove plants that I can see in bloom helps to get me up a steep hill, as it distracts me. But it also enriches the experience. I get a chance to appreciate the natural world while out running. Even if it is along a road, there is inevitably a smorgasbord of birds and street plants to see. Just being outdoors makes exercise and pain easier to bear, and we notice the effort we are making less.

I have deliberately focused on what happens to our minds while we are running because all too often the focus is on how we feel afterwards. This can put off non-runners, as they mistake the silence on the act of running for a claim that running itself feels easy. It often doesn't, and the lack of ease actually helps your mind, rather than making things worse.

But yes, many of us run with the finish in mind, rather than particularly revelling in the experience itself. We know that we will feel good, not just for the rest of the day, but for much of the ensuing week, too. The day before I wrote these words, I ran thirteen miles. For the first ten, I was with friends from my running club. I completed the final three on my own as I made my way home. My body was fatigued by this point. My legs felt like two overfilled suitcases that I had to lift repeatedly. I'd been running for enough years to know that it was fine to ignore all this physical grumbling, and so I kept going until I reached my distance. I wasn't enjoying deploying all those persuasive techniques that I listed above, but I finished. I naturally felt proud of myself. And for the rest of that day, and throughout the process of writing this particular section, I noticed that my mood was significantly better than it had been the day before. I was enjoying what some people like to call the 'runner's high'.

Why We Get High

Why does running lift our mood for an extended period of time? It can't merely be the way in which we are able to spring-clean our thoughts. What goes on in our bodies that leads to that high, or at least an improved mood?

It's reasonably well known that exercise releases some kind of chemical that makes us feel good. One theory is that the chemical is found in 'endorphins'. These hormones are released during nice activities such as sex and eating, and sometimes-nice activities like running. They increase our sense of pleasure (hence the sex bit) and reduce pain (which would explain why they appear when we run). It isn't fully understood how endorphins can alleviate the symptoms of illnesses such as depression, but then neither is it fully understood how antidepressants can have the same effect. One thing is clear, though: while running can have annoying side effects like sore knees, blisters and an inability to talk about anything other than your 5k PB, it tends to be kinder to you than many of the clunky drugs that are still prescribed today.

If my running means I don't have to take an even higher dose of sertraline, then I'm happy to end up with feet so shredded that they make my partner's daughter cry. One thing worth noting here, though, is that some medication can make running difficult. I couldn't have recovered without taking the antidepressant and sleep medicine trazodone, but equally I noticed that I just couldn't run as fast when I was on it. That's a price worth paying, but patients taking lithium have to be careful about exercising, particularly in hot weather. An imbalance of water and salt levels can exacerbate some of this medicine's side effects. Some runners with bipolar disorder also say they need to take care that running doesn't exacerbate the early symptoms of a manic phase. As ever, what matters is what works for you personally.

The high is sufficiently powerful that many clinicians use running as part of a package of treatment for patients, even those with acute conditions. We met Dr Jon Goldin when he was expressing worries about smartphones in the previous chapter: he's vice chair of the Child and Adolescent Faculty at the Royal College of Psychiatrists and is also a consultant child and adolescent psychiatrist at Great Ormond Street Hospital. He says:

Many clinicians, myself included, recommend exercise including running as part of the treatment for adolescent depression. One needs to engage the teenager and help them to see the potential benefits, which do require a degree of self-motivation... clinically I have seen the positive outcomes of exercise in teenagers on many occasions.

Running can help prevent mental illness. Research from the Karolinska Institute in Sweden found that running produces a higher level of an enzyme called kynurenine aminotransferase. This breaks down a molecule called kynurenine which has been associated with stress-induced depression, anxiety disorders and schizophrenia. Breaking down the molecule into kynurenic acid means it can't enter the brain.[6] Similarly, a 2018 study by West Michigan University found that running quickly for half an hour improves 'cortical flicker frequency' threshold, which affects our ability to process information.[7]

But running can do more than act as preventative measure for those who are healthy. It can also relieve the symptoms and lengthen the lives of those afflicted by some of the most serious conditions.

Dr Brendon Stubbs is a research physiotherapist at King's College London, and has examined the claims above. He is so convinced by what he's found that he believes physical activity should actually be a routine part of mental health treatment and placed on a par with therapy and medicines when treating conditions such as mild depression. And what he has found really is quite exciting.

Stubbs and colleagues ran a systematic review and meta-analysis of over 260,000 people who had no existing mental health problems over a seven-year period. He found that those who had higher levels of physical activity were 15 per cent less likely to develop either depressive symptoms or clinical depression in the future. This was the case for all age groups and sexes, and even when the research team adjusted statistically for other factors which may contribute to depression, they found that there was still a protective effect against the future risk of depression. For those who met government guidelines of 150 minutes of moderate physical activity per week, the risk of depression was 30 per cent less. There are similar improvements in symptoms for illnesses such as generalised anxiety disorder. But Stubbs is also very aerated about the importance of physical activity for those illnesses at the more severe end of the spectrum, such as schizophrenia. He says:

This illness can be really devastating for people. And it doesn't really get the same traction or interest from the public. But we are really concerned about people with schizophrenia because evidence has shown that they are likely to die 20 years earlier, and 70 per cent of those deaths are preventable non-communicable diseases such as diabetes, cardiovascular illness and respiratory disease.

I must admit that I was stunned when I found out why people with schizophrenia die much younger. I had assumed it was because they had a higher suicide risk. Instead, the illness leads to a number of physical health problems which are either brought on by the way someone with schizophrenia ends up living, or as a result of side effects of the medication they must take. Patients have a higher rate of smoking than the general population and they also find that their antipsychotic drugs drain them of energy while also wrecking their metabolism. In addition, people with schizophrenia experience 'diagnostic overshadowing', which means that doctors only notice their mental illness rather than the possibility that they may also have entirely separate physical conditions which also need treating. They therefore receive inferior physical healthcare screening and treatment than people without schizophrenia.

'People are dying early largely due to preventable physical conditions,' says Stubbs, with a note of disgust in his voice at the lack of attention paid to this. 'Therapy can help with mental health symptoms, but is not going to help with addressing that, and medication has, if anything, been implicated in negatively influencing physical health. It's really important that we place physical activity at the centre of mental health treatment.'

Like most other mental health problems, schizophrenia leads to a reduction in the size of the hippocampus. This is the part of the brain that deals with knowledge, memory and emotions. But Stubbs and colleagues ran a meta-analysis which found that exercise can actually increase the size of the hippocampus once again.[8] So not only can exercise keep someone alive for longer, it can also help them enjoy that life a little bit more.

Parkrun

Only a few decades ago running was considered the kind of thing
you either did if you were actually really fast or lived somewhere
like Los Angeles. And of all the movements that the policy wonks
are really fascinated with, and that has done more to change the
image of running as being a niche, elitist pursuit, you can't get much
better than parkrun.

Like many good things, this now huge global movement started
by accident. An injured athlete called Paul Sinton-Hewitt set up
a free 5k time trial in Bushy Park, Richmond in 2004. There were
thirteen runners, and three volunteers running the event. The results
were written down on paper and the finish tokens were washers
from the local hardware store. The run grew and grew, and other
runners tried to persuade Sinton-Hewitt to set up another time trial
on nearby Wimbledon Common. He was reluctant, but eventually
yielded, and a network called 'UK time trials' sprang up. In 2008,
these became known as parkruns. At the time of writing, there
are now over 5 million people taking part in these free weekly
timed events, with runs in twenty different countries. In the UK
alone, there are 600 different parkruns taking place every Saturday
morning. In England and Wales, every parkrun starts at 9 a.m. In
Scotland and Northern Ireland, runners set off at 9.30 a.m. Each
event is free and run by volunteers. And an astonishing number of
people turn up every week.

What's even more astonishing is that many of these early risers
aren't those typical runners who can swoosh their way around a

five-kilometre course with the greatest of ease. In fact, the average parkrun time is getting slower precisely because the movement is trying to encourage more people who can only walk or run very slowly. At every run that I join, there are those men at the front who seem to be a different species to the rest of us: stringy, always wearing club vests, and apparently barely fatigued after their seventeen minutes of running. But there are also families who walk the entire course, people recovering from heart attacks and strokes, and runners who have never so much as broken a sweat before, all trying to improve their time. Many – though by no means all – of the courses are wheelchair accessible. Parents are encouraged to push their children in buggies. Sport England has invested money into trying to encourage more visually impaired people to run, and local parkruns will provide volunteer guides if a runner gives them notice.

In a world that seems increasingly grumpy, with people struggling to live alongside one another particularly well, parkrun sticks out. The volunteers make as much of a fuss over the runner who staggers across the finish line after forty-five minutes as they do over the stringy character who completes the course first. There's a tail walker at every event, so it is impossible to finish last, no matter how long it takes you. In recent years, the parkrun team have tried to expand their appeal away from merely middle-class types who already find it reasonably easy to exercise and into more deprived communities. They now advertise parkrun as a 'walk, jog or run' event, and include slogans in their social media campaigns such as 'a 60-minute 5k is just as far as a 15-minute 5k'.

The UK's Royal College of General Practitioners now partners with parkrun, encouraging its members to prescribe the weekly free activity to patients suffering from a range of illnesses, whether rheumatoid arthritis, heart disease or mental health problems. There's central government funding to help parkrun reach people with long-term conditions, an online support group for park runners with mental health problems and a network of 'mental health ambassadors' who encourage healthcare professionals to refer their patients to their local run as part of their treatment plan. There are even parkruns in prisons such as HMP Haverigg in Cumbria. Prisons are generally in crisis, but wardens report that encouraging their charges to go on the run improves their mental health and the general prison environment as a result. Now, hospitals are opening parkruns too, with the Bethlem Royal Hospital the first to invite patients and locals to run together in its grounds.

One of the things that drove the focus on mental health was the deluge of stories from park runners whenever someone asked why they took part. So many of them involved people running through darkness in their soul. I have spoken to a few of those in the course of writing this book. Take Ellen Devine. Like Hope Virgo, Ellen is recovering from anorexia, and while she finds that the 'nagging voice' in her head can sound rather loud when she's exercising, she's found that parkrun is such a friendly, non-judgemental environment that she now feels more comfortable in her own skin. It has made Ellen realise that: 'I am so much more than an eating disorder.' Parkrun has meant that running isn't just about a calorie burn, but about friends, the pride of volunteering and 'being accepted'.

The benefits aren't confined to running itself, though. Jennie has always volunteered at her local parkrun ever since it started, and often led the entire event as run director. She says:

I have also completed a few runs myself, but volunteering was my niche. After a year I had a bereavement and lots of horrible issues which came out of that and a complete breakdown. I stopped going to the parkrun and became a hermit, almost, and shut myself off from the world for many months. I was in a very dark place and it's taken me a couple of years to turn that around.

But then one summer, her local parkrun was about to mark its 200th event. The volunteer team got in touch asking if she would come to the celebrations, given she had been part of the original team that had set the run up:

I discussed it over and over in my head: could I really go back? That day was a massive day in my life to walk into that park, with all the difficult memories and facing hundreds of people, some who knew me and some who didn't. I had the most amazing welcome from the team and runners alike. I felt special, needed and wanted – and this helped with the rejection issues I had suffered.

But, more recently, Jennie faced a new hurdle. Her multiple sclerosis relapsed quite seriously, and she was unable to work:

I was upset that I couldn't continue with my wonderful achievement of volunteering for the parkrun every week. Until I realised that I could be the volunteer coordinator and volunteer from my kitchen table via email.

This again has been a lifesaver for me. I am in contact with all the members of the volunteer team, the run directors, the kids that do their Duke of Edinburgh Awards, all the new volunteers, the runners who have questions and so on. I love the chats, I love seeing all the really positive feedback the team get (and dealing with the negative issues which happen occasionally) and this makes me feel included.

Being involved with parkrun has made me feel more positive about myself, and that people do need me, like me and want me. I get immense satisfaction from my contribution to so many people enjoying themselves, being happy and achieving their goals.

Abdul doesn't run at his local event at all. For him, parkrun is an opportunity to combat the loneliness he experiences as a result of his schizophrenia. Like low self-esteem, loneliness isn't a mental illness in itself, but it can lead to, exacerbate or result from mental illness. In fact, people with mental health problems are among the most socially-excluded people in the UK. Loneliness is associated with poorer physical and psychological health. Abdul recognised that he was lonely, and spent months wanting to try parkrun, before eventually making it along one Saturday morning. 'The reason I keep going is that I have the opportunity to talk to people offline,' he explains. 'It gives me something to look forward to each week. It gives me the chance to talk to people, which I don't get much opportunity to do otherwise.'

There's some research bearing out this anecdotal evidence that it's not just the physical activity that helps unwell people. Staffordshire University interviewed twenty runners suffering from mental illness in 2018 and found that parkrun was beneficial to the mental health of all of them. The study found three themes in the interviews: a 'sense of achievement', 'connecting with others' and 'it's for everyone'. Participants were particularly grateful that there were different types of volunteer role, with one telling the researchers that: 'There are volunteering posts that anyone can do, if your mental health is really bad. [If] you don't feel able to engage in tokens or timing because you don't feel able to focus at that level, you can still hold open a gate.'[9]

After a few episodes of signing up to my local parkrun as a volunteer and then pulling out on the morning because I realised I was just too unwell to leave the house, I started to warn the volunteer coordinator that I had an illness that meant I might have to pull out at the last minute. This removed the pressure of letting people down, which curiously made me even less likely to end up pulling out.

Before I was unwell, I enjoyed volunteering at what was then my local event in High Wycombe. It was where I first crossed the finish line, and I started to make friends among my fellow marshals. It wasn't the only voluntary organisation I was involved in: I was also very active in my local church. But when I moved away from the town, few in that church bothered to check I was all right, even when it became public knowledge that I was sick. My parkrun friends, meanwhile, kept in touch for years after I'd last run at Wycombe Rye. One even made the journey all the way to my new home of Barrow-in-Furness to run with me while I was on sick leave.

This isn't to say that parkrun is some kind of replacement for religion. But it does provide many of the functions that the church traditionally covered in a community. People have a sense of belonging and of being accepted despite their differences. Parkruns often collect for local food banks and link to other local charities. If you can't see yourself darkening the door of your local religious building (which I no longer can), you might find a parkrun fits the bill – and it doesn't force you to sing.

But it is not yet proven that parkrun does improve mental health. Similarly, the link between parkrun and mental well-being isn't understood. For the time being, we will just have to rely on the many people who say that it has helped them in ways that mean they keep getting up early for a run on the day of the week that most people reserve for a lie-in.

If I'm honest, I've found the 9 a.m. start impossible during the worst times of my illness. Some of the medication I was prescribed meant it took an hour to wake myself up, even with the help of double espressos. I felt sluggish for hours every morning, and the idea of dragging myself down to a cheery crowd of people and then managing to run any distance at all was just too much. While many people say that starting their Saturday with parkrun meant that even if the rest of the day was a disaster, they'd still have achieved something before 10 a.m., I considered getting out of bed a great achievement. It was only later in the day that I could start exercising.

Fortunately, for those whose pills have transformed their morning selves, Kafka-style, into slugs, there are now events starting at a more civilised time of day that combine running with mental health care. Like parkrun, Run Talk Run started as a simple weekly run in London, and has now spread around the world. Novices are actively encouraged, and the event is billed as one where it's safe to talk about mental health. Its founder Jessica Robson suffered from depression, anxiety and bulimia but hated her therapy sessions, finding that she 'clammed up' when sitting in the counsellor's room. But she noticed that she found it much easier to open up when she was running. So she set up Run Talk Run. These groups meet in the evenings, and runners are encouraged to talk to one another about why they are there and what they're going through. Friendships spring up in the way that they do in any running group, but because there is an honesty from the beginning about why someone is running, people find it easier to ask for support far earlier than they would when just making 'normal' friends.

Rebecca Toal runs the Baker Street branch of Run Talk Run. She runs to help herself recover from a number of mental illnesses, including eating disorders:

> It helps me in a number of ways. First and foremost it is the one part of the day when I'm not consumed in self-deprecating thoughts and anxieties. My mind seems to be clear and I either focus on the actual movement of running, a podcast I'm listening to or the adrenaline and runner's high that I get from exercise.
>
> Often I can act upon my newly-cleared head when I'm back from a run: for example, I'll pluck up the courage to say something to someone I've been anxious about, or I'll make a decision that I've been avoiding. I think sometimes mental illnesses can confine you to your head and so feeling tangible sensations can bring you back to reality a little. If you're struggling to breathe as a result of anxiety, the process of running can bring your breathing back into order a bit.

That's a beautifully eloquent way of explaining the benefits of running itself, but why does Rebecca think it's important to run with a group of people who want to talk about their mental health?

For her, it's about new relationships which improve her self-esteem and which get her out of the house. It's easier, she argues, to go to see people when you know you're running than just to organise to meet up for a coffee.

This is something I know well: I have spent far more time with my running group than I have with much older friends, purely because I tend to file the session away in my mind as exercise rather than a social occasion that I need to build myself up to. I often fret about whether I will perform well, even with old friends, whereas with running, the chatter comes as an afterthought.

Existing running clubs have adopted England Athletics' RunAndTalk programme, which is supported by Mind. This works with existing running clubs, including my own in Clapham, to promote mental well-being through running. Clubs hold stand-alone events, often after work rather than first thing in the morning, with a warm-up, a short run or walk and a chat afterwards. As well as providing Mental Health Champions in the club who can point members towards professional support for their problems, they also work with local mental health organisations and provide crisis contacts. These Mental Health Champions are similar to those who work with parkrun: they hold a Mental Health First Aid Training qualification and are professionals working in the field. Running really has come a long way from being a sport that involves an angry coach shouting at everyone to go faster or go home.

Wayne Singleton is one of those new-style running coaches who, far from hassling his charges to get on with it, is much more interested in encouraging them to move at their own pace. He runs a company in Cumbria called Jogging Pals, which offers couch-to-5k programmes and longer distance sessions, and is one of England Athletics' Mental Health Champions. Wayne knows why this programme is so important: in 2018 he started hearing a voice in his head telling him he needed to kill himself. 'We won the Cumbria sports award for the group of the year, and while I was accepting the award, this voice was just saying "just end it",' he says. He was treated by his local hospital's crisis care team and has had CBT. Wayne still has 'some really crap nights', but sees running as 'part of the toolbox of things that can help you'. And that's why he decided to set up something called a Mental Health Mile in his local town of Kendal.

A couple of other local towns had decided to run these events, advertised as being about the benefits to mental health of moving under your own steam – whether running, walking or pushing your wheelchair. Wayne worked out a route which meant that wheelchairs could join too and invited local runners to a pilot. He says:

It was one of the weirdest things. I didn't want it to be big, but within minutes I had someone offering their samba band for the event and the local police cadets wanted to come along too. In the end, 157 people turned up for the first one.

The overriding thing that everyone said at the end of it, whether they'd run it in a few minutes or taken two hours, was 'what a nice, inclusive event that was'. Everyone was chatting away. Everyone was smiling.

They weren't just chatting about the unseasonably good weather on that Sunday in February, but also about their own mental well-being. For Wayne, the event marked a year since he had first gone into hospital with what doctors had suspected at the time to be psychosis, but later diagnosed as anxiety and depression. He has decided to be open about his illness, and once again has been surprised by the response:

> The response has been incredible. Suddenly people were opening up to me. I don't know whether I'd just been walking around with my ears shut or something, but I had no idea how many people were struggling. I had a little note left on my chair in our office with some chocolates saying 'I can't say who I am but I've taken the decision to go to my doctor about how I'm feeling because of you.'

So Wayne has inspired people to open up about their struggles and go to the doctor about it – as well as getting more beginners into running. I expected him to be evangelical about the sport to the extent that he cannot imagine anyone not wanting to run, but that's not the case. 'Anyone can run,' he argues. 'I absolutely don't doubt that for a minute. You just have to want to do it, and not everyone wants to do it. And if you hate it, then don't do it. You'll just get miserable with exercise. Do something [else]: go fell-walking, go swimming, go cycling.'

This must be the most balanced approach I've found towards running. I am not a natural runner: if I'd been living in Kendal when I started trying to jog around the block, I would have benefitted hugely from Wayne's groups. But I know that I can run and that, with training, I can even run a marathon. What's more important to me than that is that I like running. Conversely, my partner has natural speed and stamina, but doesn't enjoy how running makes him feel. For him, the mind tunnel only appears when he's on his bike.

Pedal Power

Cycling is just better for some people. When you're on your bike, you can cover far more ground and see so much more. It gives you a feeling of freedom and control. It currently has fewer ties in popular culture to mental health than running, but there are cyclists working to change that. Sarah Strong runs a blog called 'Bikes and Brains', after finding that pedalling around the roads helps her mind work a little better. During her first episode of depression, Sarah turned to a flatmate for help. That flatmate gently encouraged her, first to visit her GP, and then to start cycling. She was a keen mountain biker and took Sarah along to help out at a local race. Sarah enjoyed it so much that she kept volunteering. After a while, she decided to have a go at racing on her own old, rigid steel bike. She says she spent most of the race being overtaken by small children but by the end felt exhilarated in a way she hadn't for a very long time.

Sarah finds in cycling the same things I find in running: she describes the 'meditative qualities of a road ride' which stop her from focusing too much on what's going on in her head and force her to notice the traffic around her. She enjoys the mixture of solitary adventures on her road bike and cycling in a group. Like most runners, she knows her bike can't cure her mental health issues. But cycling helps, a lot: 'It's rare that I'll come back from a bike ride and regret going out. The worst might be not feeling any different, but then, at the very least, I went out and did it. Something feels better than nothing.'

Runners are more likely to be forced out of their trainers by injury than cyclists, as the sport is higher-impact. But that doesn't mean that cycling is injury-free. One of the things that puts non-cyclists off is the risk of being knocked off your bike by a car. It happened to Sarah ten years ago, and the following year she shattered her collarbone when her front wheel disappeared into a pothole on a night ride:

> This was a tough time. It took a considerable time to recover from the collarbone. At the time I would go out on a club ride every Saturday and, while I couldn't cycle, I made a point of going up to the cafe to meet my friends after the ride to stay involved and not isolate myself.
>
> Feeding the social side of cycling was very important: getting together with club mates to watch races, to marshal events, helped in temporarily replacing riding with something else that was cycling-related. It reiterated that my cycling wasn't wholly about being on the bike.

Naturally, Sarah's fitness dropped as she recovered, and she found the return to cycling deeply frustrating. It was the first time she had found herself struggling to keep up with the slowest group on the club ride, 'and there were times when it felt that I'd never regain the fitness I'd had'. She slowly learned to approach cycling in a different way, looking at other reasons for going for a ride beyond her speed. She now doesn't take a cycling computer with her so that she doesn't cling to the data about how well she is doing. This is unimaginable for many cyclists, who spend much of the time when they aren't in the saddle poring over the data recorded by apps such as Strava.

But Sarah started to enjoy rides for other reasons than how many watts she was producing.

She now has a better idea of how to get through a spell of injury, or through the winter, when there are fewer hours of sunshine and the roads can be inhospitable for long rides. When speaking to Sarah about her approach to injury and fallow periods in her cycling, I was reminded of the broader struggle against mental illness: when recovery plateaus or when a relapse pops up, seemingly without warning. She says she has learned to endure those frustrating times, pushing through slowly until she comes out the other side. All of us will get injured and find it impossible to do the sport we love without a break. All of us will find our mental illnesses do not conform to the plans we've made. Part of the challenge with both is to learn to live with that.

A surprising challenge that I encountered when I started commuting by bike was other cyclists. I'd been worried mainly about drivers cutting me up or pedestrians walking out in front of me while hunched over their phones. All of those things happen with some regularity, but I was dismayed to find that a bigger irritation on the road came from the people pedalling alongside me.

Cyclists do have a certain reputation for being Lycra-clad louts who take even the most banal rides so seriously that they run red lights, shout at people on zebra crossings and swear randomly. This is largely unfair: most of us just want to get around safely and I'd wager that there are no more numpties on bikes than there are in cars or crossing the road. Some of us overreact in certain situations because we feel much more vulnerable on two wheels than we might do in a car with airbags. Others overreact on their bikes because they overreact in their offices, at home and on the train too. I have, though, observed cyclists who seem to be using their bike as a damaging form of addictive self-medication, much like drugs or alcohol. One rounded the corner at Westminster, saw tourists crossing the road and started screaming at them as though they'd just set fire to him. It was quite obvious that there was a lot more going on for this cyclist than the inconvenience of having to stop. Some cyclists I know have deleted apps on their phone that help them track their rides, as the temptation to compete with others who have taken the same route and recorded faster times becomes more powerful than the need to get to work safely and without breaking the law.

It is unfair to single out cycling in this way. People can become unhealthily obsessed with anything. Orchidelirium, for instance, pushed one of our most beautiful native plants right to the very cliff edge of extinction. It still leads to people digging up rare specimens in the countryside today (it is illegal to dig up any wild plant). Joe Harkness turned away from twitching and back to birdwatching because the obsession with chasing the latest rare specimen was making his mental health worse. Our illnesses are crafty and can seize upon things which seem wholly good, and turn them into another way of damaging our well-being. When beating someone else's time on the Embankment or possessing a plant which belongs to nature, not you, becomes more important than safety, mental hygiene and time with family and friends, then it's time to reassess whether the activities you were using to help you stay sane have gained a darker edge.

Mind Over Matter, Matter Over Mind

I only started cycling seriously when I had done so much running that my foot packed in. Things hadn't been feeling quite right for a few weeks, but, like many runners, I ignored the spreading pain in the arch of my foot, even as I ran a 10k through the streets of the Cumbrian market town of Ulverston on a hot summer's evening. It would probably wear off, I told myself, like all fools do. Then I decided that I wanted to overtake the woman in front of me in the last 200 metres, regardless of the fire in my foot. We both sprinted to the finish and pulled up in agony, she clutching her hamstring and me suddenly unable to do anything other than hobble to my car.

That thick yellow evening saw my last run for ten months. A physiotherapist diagnosed plantar fasciitis and told me to pull out of all my running commitments for the foreseeable future, including an autumn half-marathon and the London Marathon, which I had only just signed up to do for the first time for the domestic violence charity Refuge. They held the place and I sat at home, prodding my foot and wondering how I was going to stay sane. I was a month away from finishing writing my first book, an activity that is supposed to drive you mad, and I wasn't yet back at work full-time. From running four times a week – and generally at as hard a pace as I could manage – I was barely able to move fast enough to catch a bus.

I have learned a great deal about myself as I have dealt with injury. When I booked a personal trainer during my 2016 sick leave, she asked me if I was the type of person who rested an injury or who tended to run through it, hoping it would recover. I realised, as I answered her, that I was very much the latter when it came to my mental health as well as my poor weary joints. I had tried to run through the trauma that I had experienced at the start of the year, throwing myself into work, drinking more than I normally did and expecting that everything that had happened would leave no more of an impression upon me than a thumb pressed into rising dough. I'd always known, deep down, that ignoring a sore foot wasn't going to make the pain go away. Over the past few years, I've come to understand that our society's attitude to mental health problems is alarmingly similar to my foolish approach towards injuries. How many times have you been told that 'working hard is a wonderful distraction' or even that 'you just need to keep going'? Only fools would tell you to keep overloading an injury. Yet we seem to assume that our minds can take more and more pressure and never snap like a tendon.

As soon as I'd managed to clear my plantar fasciitis, I was back in my trainers and getting ready to run the 2019 London Marathon. To begin with, the training was fun. I joined a running club and enjoyed the challenge of track and tempo sessions. The long runs in groups felt easier. But in March 2019, my mental health started to wobble, after a few months of respite. I found I didn't want to be around people very much, and the thought of a 9 a.m. start to a long run in a group didn't appeal, either. I also wasn't always in London at weekends, and often found myself completing my long runs alone.

By the end of March, I was struggling, but not with injury. I'd largely kept physical niggles at bay with endless physio sessions, sports massage and a variety of bizarre-looking contraptions to roll out my tired muscles. One of them – a large massage machine with two rounded light-up bobbles on it – looked suspiciously like a sex toy, and I took to hiding it from my cleaner, just in case she got the wrong idea. But though my stiff legs weren't so bad, my mind was slowing me down. I found that the long runs required a level of mental strength that I just didn't have. To keep running, alone, for over three hours is as hard as trying to get through an intense working day when your mind isn't the full ticket. On one beautiful March day, as the apple blossom was coming out, the birds were busy nest-building and the leaves were just opening, all clean and smart, I set off for a twenty-two-mile run. I'd hoped that this would give me the confidence that I could run the full marathon. Instead, after a number of 'drinks breaks' on the Thames Path, I decided to call it quits at fifteen miles. My head just wasn't there.

We know that running can really help your mental health. We also know, by the way, that your mental health is likely to be better if you're in work. But neither of those things is always possible when you're particularly unwell. I was trying to push myself physically in a way I had accepted I just couldn't manage mentally. That week, I was on light duties for work and had pulled out of three literary festivals to promote my first book. I was struggling to motivate myself to get out of bed, have a shower and put on clothes that vaguely matched. Yet I somehow expected that I would be able to handle a twenty-two-mile run and ignore all the nagging voices telling me that I was no good. How daft.

I worked out ways of making the long runs more manageable and enjoyable. I ran with other women from my club, instead of going alone. We broke our runs down into shorter blocks, imagining on our longest twenty-one-mile training run that we only really had another six miles to go before we needed to think about the rest of the distance. With fifteen miles to go, we concluded that really, this was only two Monday night social runs and a parkrun. On that run, the three of us stopped on the Mall to take a photo together and remind ourselves that in just a few weeks' time, we'd be finishing the London Marathon on that historic road.

On 28 April 2019, I ran that marathon, and I loved every minute of it. I was used to being mocked by my friends for all the hideous mid-run gurning photos from races over the years, but the official snaps showed me beaming from start to finish. My feet bled through my trainers, and I finished about fifteen minutes slower than I'd hoped. But the endless cheers from the crowds, the silly signs and the rush of excitement on seeing my family and friends at points on the route all conspired to make me smile for longer than I have ever managed in my life before. Even in the very final throes, as I ran down Birdcage Walk with 600 metres to go, I spotted members of my local parkrun, cheering and waving a huge banner. Their photo from that moment shows me waving maniacally and grinning like a loon, surrounded by other runners who appeared spiritually broken. A few hundred metres later, I rounded the corner at Buckingham Palace and my mouth dropped open like a child at Christmas as I saw the finish line for the first time.

The high from the marathon lasted for days. Its side effects of stiff legs and swollen toes were far better than some of the annoying extras that my antidepressants have given me. But even when it faded, I retained a sense of pride in myself, that my body had been

capable of running for 26.2 miles, and that I'd managed to raise
£20,000 for Refuge while doing so.

I realised, too, that good things didn't necessarily need to be
comfortable. One of the things that seems the most off-putting to
a non-runner is how miserable runners often look when they are
in the middle of this activity that they claim to be some kind of
mental elixir. At times the marathon was very hard indeed. There
are points where you see fitter, more experienced runners pulling
up on the pavement in agony. Just over halfway, you are passed by
runners who have already reached the twenty-mile marker heading
in the opposite direction and looking tired. The London route seems
to linger for an inordinate amount of time in the docklands, to the
extent that you resent the regular glimpses you get of the glass towers
in Canary Wharf, and wonder if you'll ever finish. My pace slipped
behind what I'd trained to do, and I finished behind a man who ran
dressed as Big Ben and got trapped at the finish because his costume
was so tall. But I also found so much that was good and joyful in
that race that I ended up having one of the best days of my life.

Marathons for mentally healthy people may largely be about
mind over matter. But for someone running away from insanity,
it's often about working out how to manipulate your mind. When I
confessed to my running club my fears that, even surrounded by the
roars of the London Marathon crowd, I would find it too tempting
to stop, one of them suggested a sports psychology trick that she'd
learned. 'You should write the names of twenty-six friends and
family on your arms and think of each person as you run each mile.
Then you'll find it much harder to give up.' Given I was running for
a charity, I decided to adapt this and write a list of twenty-six reasons

why I was fundraising for Refuge. They ranged from friends of mine who had survived abuse, to aspects of Refuge's work, to women who had been murdered by their current or ex-partners.

I chose cases that I had found particularly distressing for miles that I knew would be the hardest: at Mile 21, for instance, I ran for Claire and Charlotte Hart, who had been killed by Claire's husband and Charlotte's dad a few days after they had managed to escape from years of abuse at his hands. Claire's sons Luke and Ryan spent years saving up money so they could afford to help her and their little sister get away from the man who had dominated their lives. When I met them at a Refuge fundraiser, they told me that Claire and Charlotte had only lived a few days of the life they had deserved before they were murdered. I tried to talk to them about this but found the words tripping over one another in my throat as I struggled not to burst into tears. Later, I walked to a subway and sobbed at the thought of two women only being able to enjoy a mere few days of freedom. There was no way I was going to give up running after I had dedicated that mile to them.

This trick helped me run a marathon, but it also has a wider application. It helped me break the run down into units, and helped me focus my attention away from myself. Approaching recovery from particularly bad depressive episodes or debilitating flashbacks is best broken down into something more manageable, too. When my mind has just started to work again, I rarely believe that I will be back at my desk, churning out multiple columns and agreeing to several different broadcast bids at once. But I can imagine completing the first mile of writing a short blog while at home. Perhaps the next day I may feel well enough to ring round a few

MPs and find out what is going on. After a while, returning to the office for the afternoon seems perfectly possible, in the same way as running to Mile 23 seems less daunting when you've just made it through Mile 22.

I also find it much easier to get back to working or socialising or other normal aspects of a healthy life if I'm doing it with a purpose beyond just trying to prove I am better. I'm not suggesting that I get up every morning and write noble aims for each hour on my arm, but covering a story because it has important implications for public policy is easier than feeling I have to write something simply to show my colleagues that I'm not dead. Taking a friend cold-water swimming is easier than meeting up with them for coffee, because it's less focused on how well I perform with jokes and gossip, and more on how much they'll enjoy the sensation of the water. Distracting myself with a purpose bigger than myself helps me get better, and stops me thinking about how hard it is to recover, just as my list of twenty-six reasons to run stopped me from spending too much time dwelling on that blood oozing from my feet and across my previously grey trainers.

But no matter what you have in your head during training, it isn't fair on yourself to expect that running will always make things better. And this is something that those reading this book who want to work out how to help sick friends need to remember. Yes, running can be hugely helpful. But telling someone who is struggling to just go for a run might make them feel even more useless. It might be beyond what their mind is telling them they are capable of. They might actually feel better if they go to sleep for a bit. This is why it is really important to ask people first what they find helpful, rather than prescribing your own solutions. Even if you have a mental health problem yourself, it's worth remembering that what helps you really might be totally dud for another person.

CHAPTER SIX

Cold Water That Warms the Soul

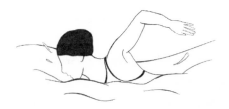

People tell me I'm 'mad' all the time. Not because of the symptoms of my illness, but because of my predilection for jumping into cold lakes in the middle of winter. Fellow journalists who've gone to some lengths to appear as understanding and supportive as possible of my mental ill health cannot stop themselves saying, 'My god, Isabel, you're mad' when I tell them I've just come from a swim in the Serpentine in Hyde Park, which was that morning covered in ice.

In truth, as I stand with one toe hovering over the cold water, I do question the life choices that led to this moment. What am I doing? Why am I about to plunge into a lake wearing only a thin swimming costume when there are people on the land wearing at least two coats? Those warmly-wrapped people aren't any wiser: one woman was so transfixed by the sight of me entering the lake on a January morning that she didn't watch where she was going and ended up slipping into the water herself.

I try not to hover over the water for too long and force myself to climb down the steps on the jetty. At first, as it washes around my legs, it feels okay. Then, all of a sudden, it really doesn't: the water hits my chest and shoulders like a slap and I gasp loudly. But then I do the maddest thing of all: I stay in that water and I start swimming. It is two degrees Celsius.

The initial shock only lasts a couple of seconds. Once you're used to it, it is strangely pleasant, like eating a little too much mustard or chewing on a strawberry bootlace. I move through the water quickly, and my body warms a little with the activity. The ice makes a ticking sound as I splash past. Sometimes, in the shallows, I pick up a broken fragment and peer through it like a window. Ducks watch me with what I've come to believe is a degree of respect for joining them in the wintry water. After a few minutes, I clamber out, skin neon and body tingling. I've submerged myself in the most powerful antidepressant I have ever encountered.

Out In the Cold

It might seem an eccentric thing to do, but cold-water swimming has been the most transformative of all the activities I have engaged in to manage my mental health. I took it up because I'd first read about the growing evidence base behind its effects on anxiety and depression. I'd come across a few cold-water swimmers who were quite evangelical about the chilling effect of the waves on their minds.

But I was not, before writing this book at least, one of those evangelists. I was generally a good girl at school, but I despised swimming and went to great lengths to avoid having to do any lengths or even widths of the pool. My sick-note forgeries were implausible but cunning. I often had periods that lasted an entire month because I knew our male swimming teacher would feel the mysteries of pubescent teenage girls to be a matter beyond his authority. On the rare occasions when I enlisted my mother in my quest to avoid the water, her genuine notes were far worse. One read, 'Isabel has been feeling rather unwell over the weekend, and I do not wish her to exert herself.'

I was an average swimmer, but rarely bothered to show that skill off. The chlorine in the school pool irritated my eczema, meaning I associated blue water with bleeding arms and red panda eyes. More than that: I had no confidence that I was any good at sport at all, something that was often flagged up in my school reports. A kindly teacher once wrote that she wished I would believe in myself a little more. A less empathetic one commented that I made no visible effort to engage in PE at all. Both were true: I didn't think I would achieve anything other than making a fool of myself either on the lacrosse pitch or in that school pool, and so I preferred to opt out.

In the years since my last mid-teen swimming lesson, the sport mysteriously became trendy. Lidos were no longer paint-peeling chilly places that swung from near-deserted to packed during rare heatwaves; instead, they became architectural and cultural gems to be appreciated year-round on Instagram. Splashing about in a muddy lake was now 'wild swimming'. If you wanted to sound fashionably sporty, you needed to be doing open-water swims to train for a triathlon. And everyone seemed to be writing a book about how the water had saved them from one trouble or another.

I found myself poring over some of these books to understand why so many people were banging on about a sport I'd spent a fair portion of my life thus far avoiding. Alexandra Heminsley writes beautifully of the way the world seemed to get smaller when she got in the water, of how free she felt, how sound disappears in the outdoors, and how she swam through the pain of struggling to conceive and miscarriage.[1] Roger Deakin, in his famous *Waterlog*, suggests that the comfort of water is because 'to swim is to experience how it was before you were born', and adds:

> Natural water has always held the magical power to cure. Somehow or other, it transmits its own self-regeneration powers to the swimmer. I can dive in with a long face and what feels like a terminal case of depression, and come out a whistling idiot. There is a feeling of absolute freedom and wildness that comes with the sheer liberation of nakedness as well as weightlessness in natural water, and it leads to a deep bond with the bathing-place.[2]

But my favourite account of swimming is a short poem by Grace Nichols, from her collection *The Fat Black Woman's Poems*. It is called 'Beauty' and describes a woman so at ease with her shape that she appears to be part of nature. It's the first poem in a collection that goes on to explore how lonely it could be to be an African-

Caribbean woman living in London in the 1980s. The Fat Black Woman struggles to find clothes that suit her, concluding that 'when it come to fashion / the choice is lean'. Meanwhile, in 'Beauty', she is found 'drifting in happy oblivion / while the sea turns back to hug her shape'.[3] The world made the woman feel uncomfortable in her own skin, whereas the water put her into 'happy oblivion'. I envied her.

Many people with mental health problems also struggle with low self-esteem, which either exacerbates their illness or develops as a result of the limitations that the illness places on someone's ability to live a normal life. It isn't so much that you don't feel comfortable in your own skin as that your skin doesn't seem to fit at all. Yet the Fat Black Woman embodies so many swimmers I have met since starting my own watery excursions. They are not the svelte 'beach-body-ready' swimmers of adverts and magazines. Instead real swimmers turn up to the sea in old skins, skins stretched over excess weight, or scarred from operations, child-rearing and all the other things that really living does to our biggest organ. But the sea turns back to hug everyone's shape. There is something beautifully equalising about the water. These days I could be swimming alongside meaty triathletes who treat the lake like a garment needing to be unzipped as fast as possible or next to an elderly woman who, even in winter, dons a straw hat to swim two slow lengths while her dogs watch from the lakeside.

Cold-water swimming is becoming steadily more popular in Britain, but there are other countries where it has long been an important part of life. Finland, for instance, has a vigorous ice-swimming culture which forms part of the country's 'Finnish spirit' or *sisu*: a courageous determination to keep going and a refusal to take the easy route. You might be more familiar with Finnish sauna culture, but that comes alongside plunges into icy water which Finns swear keeps them feeling alive and determined. Some workers take a cold dip on the way into work and as they travel home again. There are around 150,000 regular swimmers in the country and winter swimming clubs have waiting lists. Perhaps the effect of the cold water, along with the sisu emphasis on resilience, is one of the reasons Finland is regularly ranked one of the happiest countries in the world, though paradoxically, along with other Nordic countries, it does suffer from a higher suicide rate, partly as a result of its dark winters. But the possible connection between this level of happiness and the Finnish emphasis on cold water intrigued journalist Katja Pantzar so much that she wrote a book about how it – and the wider sisu – became her 'therapy' for depression which medication had struggled to fully treat. As well as lowering herself into icy water, she also met Professor Hannu Rintamäki, of the Finnish Institute of Occupational Health, who has spent years researching the effects of the Arctic climate on the body, and says cold dips cause a 'hormone storm' of mood-boosting endorphins, serotonin and oxytocin.[4]

The writing, the anecdotes and the research were all mounting, and yet I was still on dry land, just thumbing thoughtfully through more and more books. Eventually, I gave in and decided to take the plunge. My first wild dip was on a June day with Suzanna Cruickshank, who works as a professional swim guide in Cumbria, but also uses the water to keep her own mind healthy. Suzanna discovered the benefits of cold-water swimming by accident rather than design, helping her cope when caring for her father, who had terminal cancer. She didn't have time to go fell-walking, as she once had, and found herself turning to outdoor swims as a way of being outdoors while meeting her demanding caring commitments. Just a short dip in a cold lake helped her stay sane, she told me, as we walked the short distance to Grasmere.

Grasmere is small and quiet. The woods around the lakeside give the water a bottle-green colour. As I pulled my wetsuit on under a larch tree, I saw an insect called a beautiful demoiselle – a damselfly with an iridescent rich blue body and stunning black wings – fluttering around the water's edge. There were ducks. There was no chlorine. There were no shouts and squeals echoing from the roof of an over-warm pool. A fellow in a canoe was making his way over the water and, at one end, a family munched on a picnic by the shore. It was quiet. We walked in.

The water was cold, but not gaspingly-so. I'd put off cold-water swimming for so long that I would have to wait for months until I really experienced that electrifying moment when your body seizes a little on the first immersion, and then you can both see and hear your breath squeaking out of your lungs for the first few strokes. On the surface, more damselflies landed, unbothered by us in a way that was impossible on land. We chattered our way around the lake, took our wetsuits off and swam again in our costumes. This time the water felt even softer against my skin. It is a sensation I'm not sure I will ever get used to – the way the water makes me feel as though I am being held, just like Grace Nichols poetically wrote.

It was clear that swimming was something I had been missing without realising. Within days, I was a convert: I was swimming in the Irish Sea, splashing around Coniston, and changing my cycle commute in London to include a stop-off at the Serpentine.

I started to notice that swimming was particularly helping one of my most annoying responses. Many mental illnesses cause our fight or flight response, an entirely natural way of dealing with threatening situations that we can see in animals as well as ourselves, to go awry. Not only can we fail to discern what is real and what isn't, but our response to stressful events can be far out of proportion to what is really going on. Our heart rate soars, as does our blood pressure, and we can struggle to breathe.

My own fight or flight response had indeed become quite ridiculous as a result of my illness. When someone asked me to describe the overriding emotion that I felt on bad days, I thought for a while and replied that I felt frightened. Yes, I felt despair, sadness, paranoia and everything else. But the strongest symptom for me was one of utter terror at what might be about to happen. Birds take flight when they are disturbed by a noise or movement that they perceive as a threat. But the rest of the time, they're able to go about their daily lives, eating, singing impossibly loudly at one another and building nests. Of course, they're vigilant, just as we are when we cross the road to go to the shops, but I had become hyper vigilant, which is a common symptom of PTSD. I was terrified that everything presented a threat, whether I was going to the shops or having a conversation with my partner about his plans for the weekend. Wherever I looked, I found evidence that my world was about to fall apart. I often curled up into an embryonic position with fright.

On occasion, my fight response decided to make an appearance. I'm not an angry person. One of my favourite books as a teenager was *Jane Eyre*, not so much for all that 'Reader, I married him' stuff as for the way in which she learns to totally control her emotions so that no one can read her or understand her internal turmoil. I applied this very well as a young adult when a series of deeply unpleasant events took place. By the time the bad stuff was over, I'd taken quite a lot of turmoil in and shoved it into a mental cupboard. As with my attitude to housework, this turned out to be a very short-term strategy: eventually the cupboard burst open and I found myself getting inexplicably and randomly angry with people – colleagues, my partner, close friends, even a random wildlife photographer who tried to have a conversation with me about kingfishers (sorry, Phil).

Fortunately most of those people knew I was sick and understood that at some stage they'd receive a very contrite and slightly broken message from me once I'd recovered a little. But the combination of being terrified and then being utterly furious with entirely the wrong people – those who were doing the most to bear with me and support me – was making my life very difficult. It doesn't matter how often you apologise to a colleague, for instance: they still remember what you said to them and you've still made that working relationship a little less professional with your outburst. It doesn't matter how wonderfully emotionally intelligent, patient and loving your partner is: screaming outbursts, or running out of the house barefoot and into the darkness, or accusing him of hating you take a toll, and leave him exhausted and needing his own therapy. This is not a way to live. Fortunately, swimming enabled me to live better.

One July evening, I had a panic attack as I was trying to finish my work. I was in Cumbria and nothing else seemed to be working. Eventually, I drove myself to the south end of Windermere and pulled on my wetsuit. It was a soft summer night. The sun was low in the trees and the water glassy as I climbed into the River Leven, which flows out of the south side of the world-famous lake. I swam for two miles in the soft water, geese and swans flying over me, and cows watching me suspiciously from the riverbank. All I could hear was the gentle rhythmic splash of the water as I swam through it, and the occasional blackbird singing thoughtfully as the light faded.

When I arrived back at Fell Foot Park, a group swimming event was underway in the lake. The water was full of people chattering happily as they splashed about. My river swim had been quite different to the marked course that the swimmers were working their way around, but it was clear that the water had lifted all of us. The swim had helped my mind return to working order. The next day, I was well enough to work.

Summer and early-autumn swims are marvellous, as you can spend as long as you fancy in the water. I've swum along the Thames and watched a kingfisher zoom in front of my face. I've seen seals flapping about in the sea. I've lain on sun-warmed rocks and dried off after a dip in the cold waterfall plunge pools of Tongue Pot in the River Esk. This is the blissful end of outdoor swimming. But it's nothing like the transformative experience of going for a dip in winter.

It wasn't until the water temperature became significantly colder than the air around me that I understood quite how potent cold-water swimming was as a treatment. My first experience was in October. I swore loudly as I clambered down the steps at the end of the Serpentine jetty and my body hit the twelve-degree water. I swam for twenty minutes, watching the tufted ducks pootling across the water and enjoying the company of my fellow eccentric swimmers. A couple of weeks later, I felt the cold slap my lungs as, wearing a swimming costume, neoprene gloves and booties and an incongruous knitted bobble hat, I pushed off the jetty into water that was five degrees. I gasped loudly several times before starting my breaststroke, managing two one-hundred-metre lengths before hopping out. I was only in the water for seven minutes, but for the rest of the day I was a strange paradox of calmer than I'd been for a while, as well as more awake, too.

The cold became an addiction. Gradually, as I swam my way through December and January, I felt the water thicken as it neared freezing. The surface rippled more slowly as I pushed through it, the blue-and-gold light of winter sitting like a lacquer on top of the water. When the temperature dropped to a couple of degrees, ice appeared. The Serpentine swimmers break the ice on the lake every morning at 6 a.m. The Hampstead lifeguards report a queue of swimmers waiting to swim when they arrive, even in the depths of winter. My swims grew shorter, while both my bag of layers for after the swim and the size of my Thermos swelled.

The following year, I found myself longing for the ice to return to the water, watching the temperature drop with a strange glee. Winter had gone from being prohibitively cold, wet and muddy to being one of the most exciting seasons. I noticed ice crystals in the mud on the riverbank, watched kingfishers zoom over the rattling ice and marvelled at the frost picking out every detail in the reed bed.

Once I had swum in freezing water, other ordeals somehow felt more manageable. It wasn't just the good feeling that I had for the rest of the day or the fact that my arms and legs, often stiff from anxious tension, were growing suppler. It was also that I was indeed learning to control that fight or flight instinct as I learned to acclimatise to horribly cold water. My mind was more supple, too. It seemed to stretch out across the water and contract into a better shape each time I clambered back up the ladder and on to dry land. I knew, for instance, that I was capable of bouncing back from flashbacks, relapses and even incidents where someone had been unconscionably unpleasant. I also grew in my confidence. I was impressed by what my body – the body that had bunked swimming at school – could achieve. It could thrive in cold water that just the thought of would make most people shiver. It could swim across lakes, and in the sea on Christmas Day. For much of my life, I had been one of those people whose skin had never fully fitted, and yet in the winter water, in an odd-looking collection of swimwear, I was learning to feel at home in myself for the first time.

Many people struggle with their mental health in the winter. There is a condition known as seasonal affective disorder, which causes sufferers to experience far worse symptoms of depression in the colder, darker months. My illness had no seasonal patterns, but I still loathed winter because there were no orchids and my toes would turn white. Swimming changed that. It has made me delight in the cold, look forward to frosty mornings and almost resent those unseasonably warm days that appear every so often in February. When there was ice on the pavement, there would be ice in the lake, and so I was walking towards a thrilling experience. For me now, winter is a season to look forward to and savour.

How to Do It

The science of how someone is able to get into water that even has ice floating on top and, far from dying, swim on, is fascinating. Regular swimming in cold water repeatedly lowers your deep body temperature, and your brain adapts accordingly. It is quicker to constrict the vessels supplying blood to the skin, thus keeping your core warmer. Repeated immersion also leads to 'hypothermic adaptation', whereby the body learns not to shiver when in the water so that you can control your movements enough to swim. This is how someone is able to start moving through the water. Over time, you can build your resistance still further: Dr Heather Massey, who is a researcher in the Extreme Environments team at the University of Portsmouth, has found that fourteen months after the first cold-water immersions, a person still has half their cold-water shock-reduction ability.[5] This is why new cold-water swimmers can only stay in the winter water for a short amount of time compared to their more experienced peers.

My gloves, booties and hat help prolong my swims, as your extremities can really suffer in the lower temperatures. When I bought a pair of thicker swimming gloves, I was able to swim for twice as long while only wearing a normal swimming costume. But I quickly learned that it wasn't just about what I did and wore in the water that mattered. One of the biggest risks that cold-water swimmers face is not warming up properly afterwards. This then leads to something called 'after drop', when the cold blood from your extremities flows into your core and cools it, sometimes to thirty-five degrees (healthy body temperature is thirty-seven degrees). At this temperature, a person is clinically hypothermic. You can't just jump in a hot bath or sauna straight after, either, as this can make you pass out – or develop hypothermia as your brain is tricked into cooling your core when it actually needs to be kept warm. The best way to rewarm is to don as many layers as possible as quickly as possible and enjoy a hot drink.

Even though the rewarming process sounds like a bit of a bother, I soon came to see it as an important part of my regime. I would chatter with other swimmers as we dried ourselves, then take myself to a nearby bench with my Thermos, and sit in silence for five or ten minutes, watching the world go by. This was often the last bit of calm I had before a busy day at work, and the combination of a quiet few minutes alone and the euphoria induced by the cold water often enabled me to stay sane for many more hours than I would have managed otherwise. On the day that Tory MPs called a vote of no confidence in Theresa May as Tory leader, for instance, I was on the banks of the Serpentine at dawn, watching on my phone as the Prime Minister gave a statement in Downing Street. As soon as May walked away from the lectern, I clambered off the jetty, swam my lengths in the five-degree water, changed and cycled the short distance to Westminster to start a very long day. I hadn't worked a day that long or that busy for a good while. I took time to recover the next day, but I am convinced I was able to handle the twists and turns of covering that vote better because I had taken just ten minutes for a very cold swim, and five to warm up by the lakeside with a pot of porridge and a stern-looking goose keeping watch. This book largely exists because I either swam or ran every day that

I wrote it. I always regain the time I spend swimming because it means I can stay sane, alert and safe for much longer every day.

The Serpentine is a proudly spartan outdoor swimming spot. The lakeside cold shower is often warmer than the water you've clambered out of, and the tiny mixed changing room is steamy from the constant cups of tea being handed around as swimmers check that their companions can still string sentences together. One of the few rules is that you mustn't swim under the ice. There's no rule banning wetsuits, but few winter swimmers wear them: we swim for the sensation of the cold itself, not the distance.

Other swimmers advised me that I needed to stay acclimatised by swimming through the autumn as the temperature dropped, so that my body wasn't shocked by the winter water. This sport can save your life, but it has its own risks too: starting swimming in the middle of the winter is very unwise, as is swimming alone in cold weather. Some swimmers prefer to stay in groups at all times, even in the summer. I've learned to take careful precautions before going for a solo dip. No activity is without risks: fell-walkers often end up needing mountain rescue services because they have set off with a glib expectation of the day staying bright and the path being so obvious that they don't need a paper map or a compass. Outdoor swimming needs careful preparation, but you are handsomely repaid for the effort. For me, the risks of mental illness exacerbated by inactivity far outweigh the low risks of a wild dip.

The contrast between the lack of rules in wild swimming and those old-fashioned signs in indoor pools about what you must and mustn't do (including the gloriously opaque rule about 'no heavy petting', which was often accompanied by a cartoon of two people looking saucily at one another) is what attracts many people to it. Swimming in a lake, you don't have to go in straight lines. There is no one hitting your foot behind you as they catch up with you in the lane – there are no lanes! But, of course, there are rules about where you can swim and where you can't. Beyond that, there are also guidelines about where and how you might want to swim safely.

As I mentioned above, it's not a good idea to swim alone, especially not in the colder months. I often do take myself to quieter waters such as tarns or the edge of Coniston Water, but I always make sure that my partner knows where I am, when I've got in and when I've got out. I also take an inflatable tow float with me. I can store my phone and my keys safely in the centre of the float, which means I can send a GPS tracking signal to my partner to show where I am. The float itself is also luminous, as is my swimming cap, which makes me just a bit more visible in case I end up in distress. I also always take a whistle with me. Swimming in groups, I always make my own assessment of the water, even if it is an officially-organised swim. If it's the sea, I know how to recognise dangerous tides and currents, and in lakes, I always read up on the area beforehand, and check the water itself for hazards such as blue-green algae, which can be toxic and cause some very nasty illnesses. In the summer, I swim in the Thames at a historic bathing spot called Marble Hill. There are lovely steps down to the water there, and a pair of older gentlemen often paddle past in their wetsuits as I splash about. But I never swim after heavy rains, as this part of the river is downstream from a sewage works, which can overflow. I always swim at my own risk, taking my own

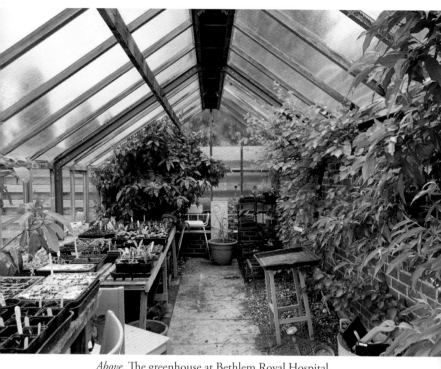

Above. The greenhouse at Bethlem Royal Hospital.

Below. Homegrown heritage tomatoes from author's garden.

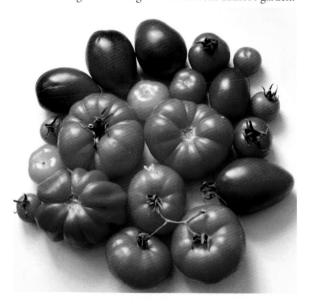

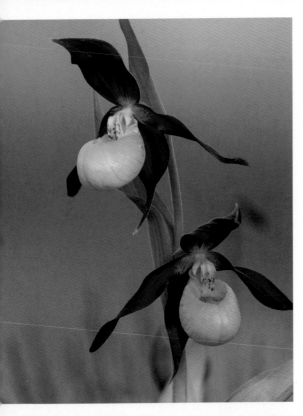

Left. Lady's Slipper Orchid, *Cypripedium calceolus*, Gait Barrows, Lancashire.

Below. A male digger wasp attempts to mate with a Fly Orchid in Kent.

Opposite top. Kingfisher with its catch near Dumfries.

Opposite below. Kestrel dust bathing in Richmond Park.

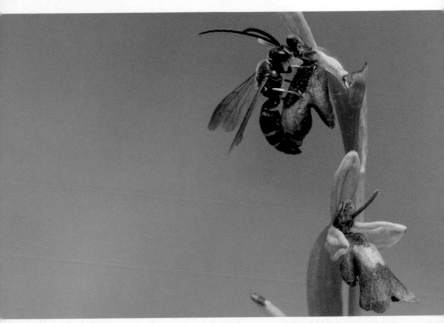

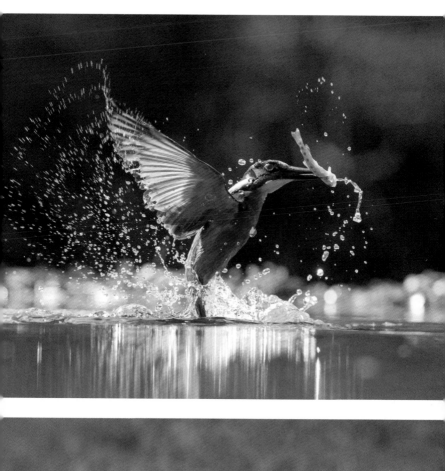
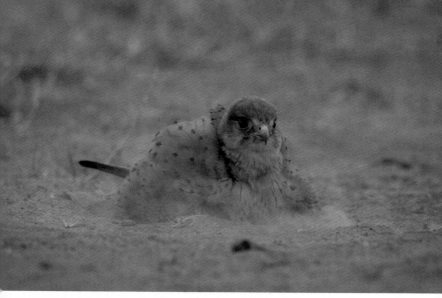

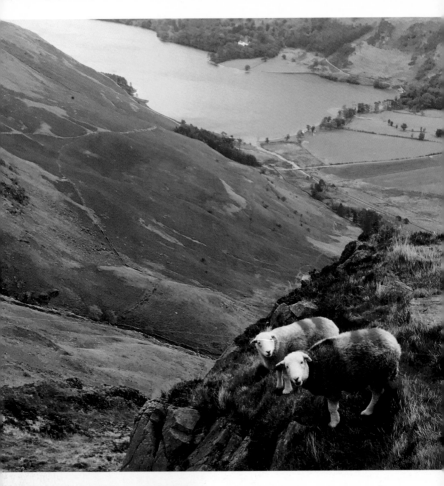

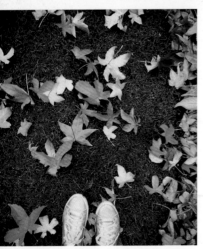

Above. Sheep on the side of Haystacks, near Buttermere, Cumbria.

Left. Liquidambar leaves in Cambridge.

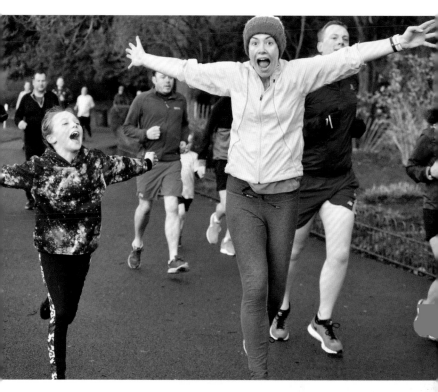

Above. Enjoying Barrow parkrun.

Right. At the finish of the 2019 London Marathon.

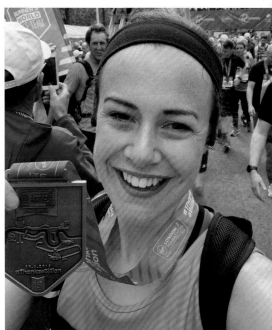

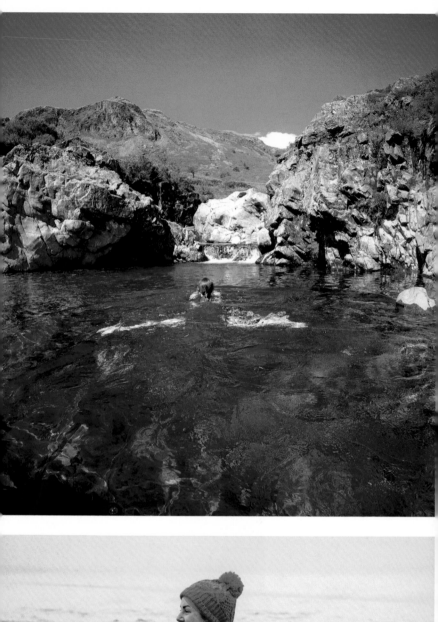
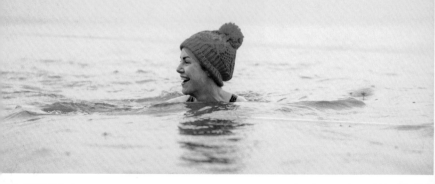

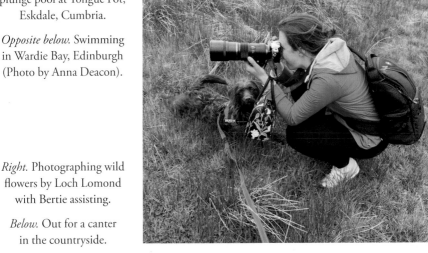

Opposite top. The waterfall plunge pool at Tongue Pot, Eskdale, Cumbria.

Opposite below. Swimming in Wardie Bay, Edinburgh (Photo by Anna Deacon).

Right. Photographing wild flowers by Loch Lomond with Bertie assisting.

Below. Out for a canter in the countryside.

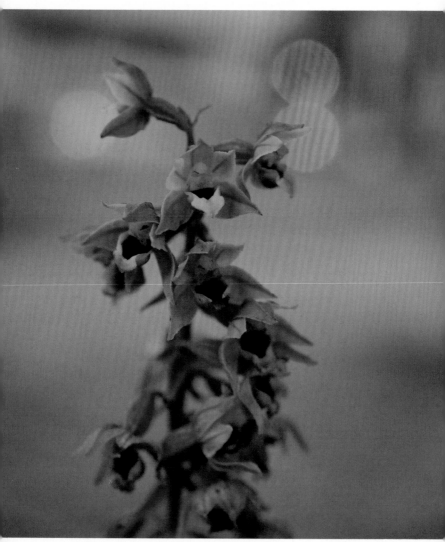

Nature can be found in strangest places: a street orchid,
Epipactis helleborine, in Glasgow.

responsibility for my safety. Sometimes, I turn up at the water's edge and decide it's safer not to go any further. In short, I try not to be daft.

Daft decisions include swimming in water that you're explicitly prohibited from entering. This might be because a landowner is nervous about health and safety, but then again it might also be because the water is a reservoir, with powerful currents and cold streams caused by dams, towers and aerators. Even if you are allowed into a lake, it may well be much chillier once you've got beyond the shallow reaches – and the shallows may suddenly shelve away, leaving you out of your depth in shockingly cold water. This is particularly the case in flooded quarries, given the way in which they are constructed. Heatwaves in Britain are often accompanied by stories of young people drowning after trying to cool off in lakes. This doesn't mean that wild swimming is a daft thing to do in and of itself, but doing so opportunistically and without carrying out the necessary research or taking the right precautions can be deadly. Always ensure that you have an easy way of leaving the water: diving in may seem graceful, but if you can't actually get out of the freezing water quickly, then don't do it.

The Outdoor Swimming Society has plenty of advice for people who want to swim safely, rather than those who are daft. It strikes a beautiful balance between evangelising about the joys of wild water and trying to advise against taking unnecessary risks. It also offers a crowdsourced map of wild-swimming spots around the United Kingdom. Some of my favourite swims, including a quiet early-autumn swim at the wonderfully named Cock Marsh on the Thames, have come from the WildSwim.com map. Swimmers set out where the best entry and exit points are, and warn about currents or hazards such as boats.

Every swimming site has its own culture. In Edinburgh, groups change under oversized coats on the breakwater overlooking Wardie Bay, trying to fend off dog walkers as their cold fingers fumble over their underwear. Lakeland swimmers take these special overcoats with them, too, teeth clattering as they chatter and share a Thermos of tea at the shore of Crummock Water. In London, the lidos might seem close together, but each has its own way of doing things. People leave the water at Tooting Bec for a stint in its sauna, talking volubly as they warm up about local theatrical productions and their theories about life. At Hampstead Ladies' Pond, the bobble-hatted women fill washing-up buckets with warm water to soak their feet in as they change back into their warm clothes. I've rarely been in the Hampstead changing room without at least one fellow swimmer walking around totally naked telling everyone how they never, ever regret making it to the water. Photography is banned when other swimmers are in the water, and every woman seems proud of what her body is capable of, regardless of what shape or size it is. The Ponds are the antidote to modern swimming-costume culture. No one cares about how taut their abs are, but instead frets about whether they are sufficiently acclimatised to swim when ice appears on the surface.

It was Hannah who introduced me to the Ladies' Pond. We met on a November morning muffled in mist. Hannah was enjoying her second winter of swimming in this strangely peaceful pool in London, and wanted to show me quite what it did for her. Like me, she had been diagnosed with something that some psychiatrists call 'complex PTSD', in her case relating to prolonged trauma in her childhood. 'I'm in my sixties now, and it's still with me,' she muttered, irritably. But then she found that the water helped it go away for just a bit. 'It's the most peaceful place in London,' Hannah explained as we shivered a little in the garden surrounding the pond. It is, and so private, too. If, like me and like Hannah, your mental illness means you can feel obsessed with whether or not you feel safe – whether in a physical location or in relationships – then this little scrap of London really is a sanctuary, even before you've stripped down to your bathers and splashed around with a bunch of ducks. It feels separate not just from the city but from the Heath too.

For Hannah, the water has an 'immediately calming' effect, even when she has left the house feeling dreadful. She then finds herself on a high as she walks away from the pond down the wooded lane that leads across the Heath and back to the world. 'I feel motivated, and wanting to get on with the day,' she explains. 'That was unthinkable before.' It has also helped her with a serious physical health problem that is made far worse by colds. 'Last winter I didn't have a single cold. And I feel stronger in myself, too, because I have become physically stronger and fitter.'

Hannah says swimming has been 'transformative'. Whether I am soaking my cold feet in the washing-up bowls by the Ladies' Pond, shivering by Buttermere in Cumbria or nattering in Wardie Bay, I hear that word from almost every swimmer I meet. For example, Lucy is in her early twenties and works as an accountant in the south of England. She swims in the sea. She, too, says the experience has been 'transformative' for the psychosis, depression and anxiety that she has required hospital treatment for over the past four years:

It's calming. When I'm swimming, I'm not really thinking about anything else. I'm not really thinking about the psychosis and what could happen. I feel a lot calmer for a couple of days after, too. My head just feels purer. I suffer from a lot of panic attacks but I don't tend to get them for a couple of days when I've been swimming.

Gaynor was so unwell during her first bout of severe mental illness that she believed a nuclear bomb had been dropped on London. She spent three months in hospital and has been sectioned on four occasions since. Her health is now stable and she says that, along with a 'wonderful' supportive partner, cold-water swimming has been a major factor in her recovery:

The benefits were amazing. From my first attempts I felt an amazing relief. I felt brave and almost invincible. When I enter a very cold lake in a wild place the world is still. It is only me and the water. The freezing-cold water silences any chattering thoughts. All there is is my physical being and the fight to overcome the cold, to master it, to survive the water. The water makes me produce inner strength to combat the physical. The cold tells you to stand still, but my control commands me to swim, dive, move.

One strange side effect of outdoor swimming was that I found a hobby to keep me happy indoors as well. I had taken to wearing brightly-coloured bobble hats to keep my head a little warmer on particularly icy days. One day, I spotted a woman in Richmond Park wearing a ludicrously lurid hat, with sky-blue and yellow stripes, and a bright pink pom-pom. I wanted a hat like that, I decided, and set about learning to knit it. One of my oldest and loveliest friends,

Fiona, is a knitter. Almost every time I visit her, she produces a hat or a scarf that she's whisked up for me. I'd noticed that she seemed so very content when knitting, and she told me that it made her feel the most in control that it was possible to be as a mother of two young children. She recommended a beginners' knitting book, and I set to work. Within a fortnight, I'd made my first bobble hat.

I realised that the methodical actions of knitting, purling, slipping a stitch and making another kept my mind from whirring too much. Oddly, it made me better able to focus on things, and I often secretively knitted while watching late parliamentary debates and political TV shows, as I took more in. It satisfied the smoker's twitch that I'd developed towards my mobile phone, meaning that my screen time plummeted by a third within a few weeks. On long winter evenings and train journeys, I found something productive to do that stopped me scrolling through the social media feeds of people who were not mentally ill and whose apparent success and good health I therefore envied bitterly (even if well-curated social media was in fact masking what was really going on in their own lives). I now own more bobble hats, jumpers and scarves than is probably decent. But at least I'm always the warmest swimmer by the lakeside.

Many swimmers, including Lucy, Hannah and myself, need medication and therapy alongside their swimming, but for some patients, swimming is enough to help them stop taking the drugs they were originally prescribed. Sidney has bipolar disorder and PTSD, and gained so much weight when being treated for the former that at one point he was thirty stone. He is a veteran with physical and mental injuries from his service in the army and special forces, but government cuts to his respite care left him without the support he needed. He learned how to swim front crawl in a way that didn't exacerbate the damage to his shoulders and knees, and now swims in his local docks four or five times a week. 'The only thing I'm worried about is my next stroke and my next breath,' he tells me. 'I don't have any worries at all. It replaces medication for me. It allows clarity when I get out. I feel more of my natural self.'

There are downsides, though. Sidney has noticed that he can end up 'buzzing a bit too much' after a cold swim, which is a warning sign for bipolar patients that they might be on the verge of a manic phase. 'I have to calm myself down a bit and plan things day by day,' he says. 'Otherwise I'll be planning an £800 swim in Greece and planning all these big things when what I need is to just focus on what I'm doing in my next local swim.' There is some evidence that intense exercise such as running can be unhelpful to bipolar sufferers who are on the cusp of a manic phase. The same may well be true of cold-water swimming, as it could overly energise an already overexcited mind. One sufferer who I spoke to during the research for this book tried cold-water swimming when he was on the verge of mania. He felt it helped him, but his condition worsened and he was sectioned a little later. It could have been that swimming did help a bit and that the onset of his symptoms was inevitable. But it's always important to talk to your doctor about what will and won't work – and to keep an eye on the effects of new activities, just as you would with medication.

Exercise is good for the soul, but all good things are best in moderation. Neil Cooper found this as he tried to manage the

PTSD he developed as a result of his work as a police officer and his service in Kosovo. He says:

> I think I've been to triple figures of post-mortems including child and baby deaths. And despite my belief otherwise for many years, your brain can only cope with so much. I got to the point of burnout, but was trying to hide it away and soldier on. I had insomnia but was working non-stop, and found family life very hard to cope with.
>
> Eventually it got to the point where nothing worked any more. I took up triathlon and the worse I got, the more obsessed I got with that. I knew I was in trouble because I was going out on my bike and the harder I pushed myself the worse I got. I saw a professional and they said, 'You've got to start doing things more gently because this obsession with trying to hurt yourself isn't working.'
>
> The only place I would actually get peace would be on a Friday night in Ullswater or Derwentwater, in the middle of those lakes in the night. The open water is something that has helped me. I'm not worried about my pace or time, it's just getting out into the lake for the peace, the quiet, the views.

Ullswater is the second largest lake in the Lake District and has an inky magnificence to it at dusk that helps even a screaming soul calm down. I have floated in the middle of the lake filing my thoughts neatly away on many an evening. And as I've swum there and in rivers, ponds and lidos across the country, I've found myself wondering more and more why something this transformative isn't getting even more attention.

Why It Works

Fortunately, the medical world is starting to take a better look, moving from the hunch that we've had since Roman times that water might be a good thing to a desire to understand what's going on and who might benefit from a dip. Researchers have discovered many possible physical benefits that go far beyond general fitness: there is some work which suggests there might be a link between cold water and a stronger immune system.[6]

The outdoor swimming community is awash with near-evangelical beliefs about the benefits of the water, and not just for the soul. Some swimmers extrapolate research suggesting that cold water can improve your immune system into an assertion that you never get colds if you keep going through the winter. My first winter season did pass without a single cold, it is true, but I know many swimmers who have had to take time off from the water because they have gone down with the kind of stinking bug that everyone gets from time to time. There is, though, a theory that the stress reaction caused by entering cold water could stimulate the production of white blood cells, which are a key part of the immune system. And it's not just our ability to fight off a cold or our mental health that apparently benefit. A half-serious survey of swimmers at Tooting Bec Lido reported more than a quarter claiming that a dip was almost as good as an orgasm, which raises a number of questions unrelated to the sensation of breaststroke.[7]

An increasingly fashionable movement concerned with the health benefits of freezing yourself silly is the Wim Hof Method.

Its proponents claim that it can suppress inflammation, as well as improve sleep and lower stress. It can even help people cope with depression, they say. A mixture of meditation, breathing exercises and exposure to the cold, it was developed by a Dutch man called (funnily enough) Wim Hof. He has climbed Mount Everest in his shorts, and stood covered in ice cubes for more than an hour. These feats make taking a dip in a chilly English lake seem a bit tame. They also sound impossible and dangerous.

Yet research into the Wim Hof Method has led to some scientists reconsidering aspects of immunology: in 2012, the Radboud University Medical Centre in the Netherlands studied Wim Hof to understand how he could manage to spend so much time around ice and stay alive, let alone comfortable. They discovered that his technique actually calmed down his immune system so that it didn't overreact to a simulation of a sepsis that they had created. He was also able to control his autonomous nervous system, which controls our heartbeat, blood flow and so on. To check that Hof wasn't just a freak of nature, the scientists then trained a group of volunteers for fourteen days and made them perform the same experiment. Those volunteers had the same response.[8] It's worth noting, though, that there was no placebo group in this study, and it didn't examine the long-term effects of the method, either. I wouldn't start running naked up mountains just yet.

Some aspects of the method are commonly accepted as being helpful for lowering stress levels, such as breathing techniques. Others sound, well, a bit dodgy. Hof claims that he can change the pH of the blood to a more alkaline state, which is good for our well-being. There's no science to back that up.

Let's take a look at where accepted scientific research is heading on cold water and more widely on the causes of some mental illnesses. It's fair to say that scientists haven't moved on much in understanding the drivers of these conditions over the past few decades, but more recently, the psychiatric world has started to take note of a new theory, which is that depression could be caused by inflammation. One of the leading practitioners of this theory is Professor Edward Bullmore from the University of Cambridge, who has investigated the link between the immune system and mental health. In his book *The Inflamed Mind*, he explains that when we are stressed, whether physically or mentally, our bodies release inflammatory proteins called cytokines into the blood.[9] These then cross the blood–brain barrier and cause the brain to become inflamed. It's not fully clear what happens after that, but what sparked Bullmore's interest in the first place was that a patient he saw many years ago with the inflammatory disease rheumatoid arthritis was also depressed. His colleagues at the time dismissed his interest in this, pointing out that anyone with that debilitating condition would end up depressed. But Bullmore now believes that this patient was depressed as a result of the same inflammation that was causing her physical illness.

He also notes that certain medicines for physical illnesses have a curious impact on mental health. An inflammatory drug called interferon, for instance, treats hepatitis B, but also makes the patient clinically depressed. Could the inflammation that the drug is supposed to cause in the patient also be causing their depression? Then there's the 'Remicade high', which swiftly follows the administration of a treatment for rheumatoid arthritis. Patients suddenly become extremely happy after receiving it. Could this be more than a coincidence? As with everything mental-health-related, there is so much more research that needs to be done before the shift in treatment that Bullmore predicts will actually happen. But that research is at least underway.

The leading physician researching cold-water swimming and mental health in the UK is Dr Mark Harper, who became interested in the way cold water warms the soul after he took up swimming in the sea in Brighton in the winter. He was struck by how exhilarated he felt after each dip, and set to work examining what could be going on. Studies had already established that repeated immersion in cold water was able to diminish the fight or flight response.

A 1988 study found that as few as four repeated immersions in cold water can help people to control that fight or flight response.[10] Then in 1994, researchers in Berlin found that regular swimming in ice-cold water during the winter increased people's tolerance of stress by decreasing the concentration of uric acid – which is linked to inflammation – in their plasma.[11] Scientists in Washington made people sit in cold water for fifteen minutes in 2002, which you might expect would stress anyone out, but instead it decreased their heart rate by almost 10 per cent and reduced their blood pressure. Participants also reported feeling calmer.[12] A similar study in Prague in 2000 asked a group of young men to sit in water of various temperatures. At fourteen degrees Celsius, these men saw levels of their dopamine increase by 250 per cent.[13] Dopamine is a chemical that influences the brain's pleasure and reward centres, and is believed (that lack of certainty right there, again) to play a part in treating depression. So if raised levels of dopamine could improve depressive symptoms and cold water caused a significant increase in those levels, then it follows that cold-water swimming might have an antidepressant effect not dissimilar to the way medication influences our serotonin receptors.

Harper wanted to find out whether the underlying cause of an overactive fight or flight reaction could also be treated using cold-water swimming. First, he had a go with one patient, who also rather bravely agreed to be featured on a BBC One programme, *The Doctor Who Gave Up Drugs*.[14] This patient had been taking antidepressants for eight years, but has since stopped as a result of the transformation in her symptoms that swimming brought about. She still has a diagnosis of depression, but manages it instead by swimming in a local lake.

When someone first gets into the water, Harper explains, the shock of the cold will be such that they won't be able to control their breathing. It will feel just like a panic attack. But then, slowly, they'll be able to get their breathing back under control. Then they'll be able to swim. 'Within six swims, you will be adapted to cold water.' Then, he suspects, any mental illness associated with stress and inflammation, including depression, generalised anxiety disorder and PTSD, could see its symptoms alleviated by cold water.

The next step was to set up a course that started people off swimming in a pool, before taking them out into the sea once they were sufficiently confident. The research is still ongoing, but the anecdotal reports so far are that the swimmers' mental health has improved.

It's easy to find anecdotes of swimmers whose lives have improved immeasurably as a result of cold water. I'm one of them. But the more lakes, rivers and lidos that I splash about in, the more I wish there was a way I could argue convincingly for the benefits of a dip without resorting to 'It worked for me'. What if proper research does conclude that cold-water swimming, often considered the preserve of the mad, might help people stay sane? What if it reduces the need for some patients to take medication which can cause physical health problems that can even shorten lives? We don't know yet if those things are true, but there is a compelling case for the medical world to dive in and find out more.

—

CHAPTER SEVEN

All Creatures Great and Sane

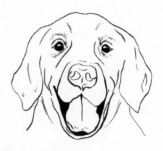

Fudge is a chocolate Labrador. She's just an ordinary dog, who pulls the same ecstatic face when she's about to roll in fox poo as any other hound. But Fudge has also saved lives, just by going about her everyday business. Her owner, Craig MacLellan, is a former soldier who developed PTSD as a result of his time serving in the Royal Marines and the Scots Guards. He left the military of his own accord, and at first found success in a new career in IT. But things fell apart. 'I didn't see anything coming. I didn't see the signs,' he explains. 'I became a workaholic and one day I woke up and I just broke down. I didn't have a clue what was going on. All of a sudden I couldn't cope any more.'

His doctor's initial diagnosis was that Craig was stressed. It took another two years before the NHS worked out that his military background might have more to do with what was going on. Eventually, he found his way to veterans' charity Combat Stress, and started getting help. But, in the meantime, Craig had stopped working, and barely left the house:

> I couldn't face the world. I ended up not being able to go out during the day. I've got a very supportive and loving wife and, despite all her efforts, she didn't know what to do either. I got to the stage where I only went out at night with the dogs. I walked in the countryside across fields purely and simply so I could avoid the world.
>
> The one constant I had were the dogs. It was that simple companionship: not having to explain yourself, a dog coming up and giving you a wet nose and a wag of the tail.

As he started getting help, Craig took his dog along with him to therapy. He asked if he could bring her along to a six-week residential run by Combat Stress. His therapist agreed that Fudge could join for the first three weeks, during which time they would work on weaning Craig off depending on the dog. But in the end, Fudge stayed the full course. She ended up helping not just her owner, but all sixteen veterans who had come along too.

No one really realised what was happening to begin with. Fudge was supposed to sit quietly behind Craig's chair during group therapy, but instead she wandered around the whole group and chose to sit with another person. It seemed initially like the kind of thing a dog will do: all of them like to shuffle and fidget about when they're bored. But gradually, everyone in the group began to notice that Fudge was up to a bit more than plodding aimlessly around. Craig says:

> What we started to see was she was homing in on whoever seemed to be the most anxious. Likewise if guys would get upset, she would just sit with them within arm's reach so they could touch her. They told me that this was helping them, it was soothing them. She brought the whole room to a basic level with everybody. She wasn't judgemental and the guys recognised that.

> We just kind of thought it was cute. But as time went on, as we walked up and down the corridors, she would sit outside someone's room. She's waiting for treats, I thought, and then we would find out that there was a guy in the room who was having a bit of a meltdown. They always wanted her to go in, and I would leave her there. Rather than the guy being in the room for the rest of the day, maybe ten minutes later he would come back out and bring her back to me and say: 'She knew I wasn't right.' They were pleased that my daft chocolate Labrador was going in and wagging her tail and trying to help.

After three weeks, Craig was supposed to take Fudge home. 'But the guys mutinied. They said "No way is she going back".' So she stayed. And by the end of the course, Craig had a feeling that he might be on to something about dogs and mental illness. The other veterans agreed.

Craig set up a charity called Veterans with Dogs, which now provides registered assistance dogs to ex-military personnel suffering from mental illness. He assembled a team of professionals in the fields of psychology, dog behaviourism and so on, and researched how other countries look after their distressed veterans. He learned as much about what not to do as about what he could copy: in the United States, for instance, Craig found that assistance dogs were being trained to defend their owners, which is ethically problematic to say the very least. By contrast, the Veterans with Dogs training involves a veteran being carefully vetted to ensure they are in recovery, that they have recognised their illness and that they are able to look after a dog, before being matched with one of three breeds: Labrador, retriever or spaniel. This is because these types of dog have been bred not just to retrieve, which comes in handy as we shall see, but also because they are naturally eager to please.

Trained assistance dogs can do the most extraordinary things. One of the charity's clients claims to have a dog who can warn her forty-eight hours in advance of her having a psychotic episode. This means that she can get home to where she is safe and get her emergency medication ready. Others bring their owner's medicines to them every day so that they don't forget to take them. Some can seemingly sense when a veteran is about to have a night terror, and either wake them up or snuggle alongside them to comfort them.

Although such feats might sound fantastical, they shouldn't come as a surprise: not only are dogs well known for being able to sniff out bombs and drugs, they are also recognised for being able to tell when their epileptic owners might be about to have a seizure.[1] Some are trained to find tumours in humans. It is hardly a stretch to understand that a dog can also detect emotional changes in their owner that are so subtle even a family member might accidentally overlook them. The bond between a normal family dog and their owner is strong: the rather cheesy saying 'man's best friend' does have a pretty strong foundation. But a trained dog for a veteran really can save lives.

Craig also explains that the dogs help their owners manage their symptoms better, which means that, over time, they may have fewer acute phases of their illnesses. Some only ever need one assistance dog and don't take on another one when the first retires at around eight to ten years of age. Others always need a bit of help from a hairy friend.

Since he set up the charity, Craig has been surprised by what he's learned about the relationship between dogs, their veterans and their wider families. In some cases, a client's partner will become jealous of the dog because the veteran will no longer rely on their human companionship so much. It's a shock to them and a loss of identity when that person starts to get better and more independent. The charity has also had to work out how to deal with bereavement, as dogs don't live as long as their owners:

> With PTSD we are generally dealing with a sense of loss of some kind. Our guys are dealing with the loss of identity from leaving the military, or a feeling of being rejected by their country. They may have lost someone while serving. When the dogs retire from doing the assistance work, they stay with their owners to prevent that sense of loss but we have bereavement processes in place so we can treat it as a normal stage of life, rather than something that causes another mental health crisis.

Another thing that shocked him was the way the public treat assistance dogs. All the Veterans with Dogs animals wear special jackets showing that they are assistance dogs. 'They're like a magnet for people. You get people crossing the road to talk to you, and they say the stupidest things. People will say "Oh, you have an assistance dog, what's wrong with you?" or "Oh you were in the army, so how many people have you killed?"'

Initially I am stunned by this. How can anyone think it is sensitive to accost someone who needs an assistance dog and ask them to dredge up the very reasons for having the creature, just for the entertainment of a stranger? But then I think about some of the foolish questions ostensibly wise people have asked me about the reason I have PTSD. I suspect I've also asked many people with mental health problems similarly idiotic things without even realising – even during the course of writing this book. Fortunately, the charity decided to make it easier for the veterans to get through these encounters without having to tell the stranger to sod off: they now carry business cards which explain that they are busy working with their dog and cannot stop, and directing the person to the website to find out more about the work of the charity.

The veterans also need training on how to deal with another type of confrontation, which is when they are somewhere that only allows registered assistance dogs. Staff in public gardens or properties can sometimes be totally insensitive to someone with an assistance dog, demanding in a rather officious way to see documentation without thinking about the effect it might have on the dog's owner. I witnessed one example of this a few years ago while visiting a famous garden which only allows registered assistance dogs. A group of gardeners accosted a man who was walking through the rockery with his animal and told him that dogs weren't allowed on the site. This seemed strange given all visitors have to pass staff to enter the garden. There was no way this man would have got his dog in without permission anyway, and now he was being accused of letting his mutt ruin the plants (it wasn't: it was sitting quietly at his feet, something trained assistance dogs must be able to do). The man's reaction seemed, to those around him, totally over the top. He became very angry and emotional and shouted that he had already been through this with the team on the gate. He produced the documentation showing that he had a legal right to bring his dog with him. The gardeners moved on, but the man was so visibly shaken by the encounter that he sat on a bench, hunched up and emotional.

Given the relationship between humans and dogs throughout their shared history, it's hardly a surprise that these creatures can help with therapy as well as herding sheep, burrowing to catch badgers or retrieving the spoils of a shooting expedition. We have long bred and trained dogs to make our lives easier – and in many cases to be our friends. Our belief that they can help us with pretty much anything is clear across the world. In European countries including Germany, Austria and Switzerland, some head teachers allow dogs in classrooms as they believe the presence of an animal calms the children down and encourages them not to make so much noise. Studies on the impact of 'school dogs' are limited, but what research there is found that children were indeed less likely to show aggression in the classroom, that preschoolers found it easier to concentrate and that children had a better attitude towards school and learning as a result of a dog being present.[2]

I don't have an assistance dog: I have a daft Labradoodle called Bertie who we'll meet shortly. But I did understand what was going on for this man in the rockery. I don't know why he needed his dog, whether he was a veteran or whether the animal was trained to detect a seizure. But he had been humiliated and his need for a pet that was probably keeping him alive and safe every single day had been questioned. If he did have PTSD, then he would have struggled with the same uncontrollable anger and shame that I know all too painfully. His day had been totally ruined, and it probably would have taken several days more for his mind and his body to recover from the stress caused in just five minutes.

Craig was worried about the problems with anger when he started trying to match dogs to veterans. It is a feature for all sufferers of PTSD, but what marks out ex-military personnel is that they have the ability to exact their anger in a particularly effective way. What if they took their feelings out on their dogs? While the charity has had to take dogs away from a couple of veterans who haven't been able to look after them properly, it has found that the pets have actually diminished the feelings of anger and allowed clients to start to deal with their emotions properly. 'They can allow themselves to love a dog because it doesn't have all the human connotations of a relationship.'

Bertie and Other Animals

How can a dog be so good at teaching a human to love and trust again? It sounds daft, almost bordering on the sort of thing you'd hear from someone who owns too many cats. But then again, it works. There's evidence that it works not just with dogs but with other animals too, who have a natural ability to help our minds.

A 2014 review suggested animal-assisted therapies might help with depression, schizophrenia and addictions.[3] Another systematic review of forty-nine studies in 2007 found that therapy animals could improve symptoms and life quality for people with autism, behavioural problems and issues with emotional well-being.[4] Similarly, a 2019 study of assistance dogs in Australia reported a range of breeds helping with depression, PTSD, bipolar and schizophrenia.[5]

In 2018, the Centre for Mental Health published a report suggesting that therapy dogs could reduce the risk of self-harm among prisoners.[6] Rethink Mental Illness ran a pilot therapy dog scheme in three prisons in the north-east of England, and found that contact between the animals and prisoners led to 'a marked improvement in wellbeing and a marked reduction in the severity of need'. The dogs also helped some of the men and women they worked with talk about problems they might normally struggle to articulate.[7] In 2012, the Mental Health Foundation looked at whether cats can help with mental well-being, too, carrying out a survey with the Cats Protection League which found that 87 per cent of people who owned a cat said it had a positive effect on their well-being and 76 per cent said they could cope with everyday life much better.[8]

Everyday life is generally much more joyful when there are animals around, it's true – unless they misbehave. Like Fudge, my dog Bertie loves fox poo. There is nothing more disgusting-smelling than this stuff. There is also, according to a dog, nothing more delightful. Bertie is a boisterous, happy-go-lucky soul, but he is never happier than when he is just dropping his shoulder, ready to smear his head and torso in a pile of excrement. I almost feel bad that I'm stopping him from enjoying what he seems to view as a luxury spa experience. But then again, fox poo stinks, and I only have so much time in the day for hosing the little scamp down in the back garden while swearing volubly.

I got Bertie because I fell in love with him when I met him at his breeder's home while camping (and writing this book), rather than because a doctor told me to. Many people had contacted me when I was researching what helped with mental illness, and before I'd thought of getting a dog of my own, to tell me that their pets had saved their lives. But, even though I've always had cats and other pets, I was a bit sceptical.

However, since having my own daft pooch, I've realised quite how empathetic dogs can be. Yes, Bertie ignores my deeply-held feelings about fox poo, but he is also aware of changes in my demeanour, and seems to respond accordingly. When I am so depressed that I struggle to get off the sofa, he plods quietly around me, licking my face every so often to check I am okay. Indeed, he is always checking that *everyone* in the family is okay: if one of the children cries, he runs up to comfort them. If my partner is low and withdrawn, he jumps on to the sofa beside him, lets out a puffing sigh from his wet brown nose and snuggles quietly with him. When I go swimming, Bertie stays at the water's edge (he's daft, but he's too sensible to think that freezing water is a wise option), watching intently to ensure that I am safe. On a train journey, he spotted that a woman opposite us was growing steadily more distressed about an argument she was having with her (soon-to-be ex-) boyfriend by text message, and shuffled over to place a paw on her knee.

He's no Lassie, but he's pretty handy to have around as a pal. But for me, the best thing about my dog is not so much his emotional intelligence as his insistence on a daily walk.

Before this scruffy creature turned up in my life, I thought I was pretty good at getting outdoors. Hell, I'd even signed a contract to write a whole book on the thing. But there were days when I didn't leave the house, and when I felt that staring at my houseplants and giving them a bit too much water was a reasonable substitute. This is naturally not acceptable to Bertie. He does not see the point of houseplants, especially not now he has been trained not to urinate on them. For him, the only possible reason I could be getting up each morning is to take him for a walk. Even as I shuffle miserably about the kitchen, Bertie is picking up my wellies to tell me that the deadline for the walk is swiftly approaching. His delight on seeing his lead and a tennis ball appear sometimes feels as powerful as the antidepressants I've just knocked down my throat.

Bertie means that before any sort of day has started – whether busy with work or heavy with illness – I've got up and have been in the great outdoors for at least half an hour. His daft smile and delight on approaching the park makes it harder for me to feel totally desperate. He makes me laugh more every single day. No, I don't get to the end of a walk and realise my frantic thoughts have gone, or discover that I am able to write sentences. But I do feel just a little more positive about being alive.

Dogs manage this so effortlessly. One woman I met told me that her husband, suffering from a terminal illness, didn't get out of bed for months before they got a puppy. But the big appealing eyes of a dog pulled him out from under the covers and downstairs to feed him. My friend Rachel, who suffers from cystic fibrosis, has a rescue dog called Rebel. Rachel suffers from all the pain and limitations that this illness causes people in their thirties, as well as the mental health troubles that are very common for sufferers whose life expectancy hovers over them threateningly. 'Sometimes I can't face getting up at all,' she says. 'But then I do because I just want to make everything okay for Rebel.'

Why do dogs manage to get us out of bed when our partners can't? It's not surprising that some of the spouses that Veterans with Dogs meets have trouble adjusting to the new family member: it seems rather unfair that a creature that rolls in fox poo can really help that much. Everyone who appreciates their dog says the same thing: it's the simplicity. Yes, a dog needs you to feed her and take her out for a walk and a toilet visit. But she doesn't need you to offer amazing chat, to do the dishes or to produce an impressive presentation at work. Her devotion isn't predicated on how much of an interest you take in how her day has gone, or your ability to swallow all your feelings and pretend that everything is okay. It is easy to feel you are letting a human down. It is far harder to disappoint a dog (except when you refuse to let them roll in a pile of poo).

Riding the Black Horse

Bertie's simple demands have taught me a lot about myself. But another animal has taught me far more. Penny Black is a cob pony, with a dark brown coat and the delightful twirling moustache that cob-type horses grow. She lives in Richmond Park at a stables called

Holly Lodge. When I first met her, she was introduced to me as a 'schoolmistress', which in horsey parlance is the type of steed that teaches the rider more than the rider can teach the horse. I naturally thought this referred to her reliability as a mount, but it turned out that her most erratic behaviour taught me the most valuable lesson of all.

Penny Black is a mare. If you don't know much about horses, you might assume that stallions (uncastrated male horses) are the challenging ones because of all the hormones raging around them. This can be true, depending on the breed, but what is universally true is that mares tend to live up to the use of their name as an insult. They can be complete nightmares.

Any woman who feels she has particularly bad premenstrual tension should spend some time with a mare coming into season to realise that human mood swings really are pretty mild compared to the equine equivalent. I discovered this the hard way. I'd been riding since I was eight years old, and I thought I knew Penny well enough by now. When I arrived at Holly Lodge, I was looking forward to grooming her, tacking her up and then a cheery ride around the rolling landscape of Richmond Park. The horse I led out of her loose box, though, was quite a different beast to the one I'd ridden a week previously. She seemed intent upon stamping on my foot as I groomed her. She tried to back me against a wall when I brought her saddle out. And when I was mounted, she pranced about the yard in an excited, jittery fashion.

Out in the park, Penny was hypervigilant. Her nostrils flared and she continued to dance around. Everyday hazards, like the noisy cyclists who throng around the roads, seemed to annoy her disproportionately. One group of bikes came a bit too close and she did a half rear. I just about stayed on. But a few minutes later, a piece of machinery parked by the track gave her the perfect excuse to do what she'd been intending to do all along. Penny threw me off, twisting as she did so, sending me flying into the soft bracken, and cantered off. Eventually we caught her, and I obeyed the age-old rule of getting straight back on the horse. But I wasn't happy. I rode her back to the stables, Penny still snorting and jittering. Already weeping, I untacked her and went on to my next appointment, which was a group therapy session run by a charity in another part of London.

The following week, I found I had too much work on to make it up to the stables, so I sent my apologies. The week after that, I was away. And then the week after that, I had no excuse, but didn't make it anyway. I was paying to ride a horse once a week, but wasn't actually riding her. This wasn't even the first time I'd fallen off a horse; it would be impossible to have ridden for so many years and not have had a few spills along the way. The difference this time was that I had been sick, really sick. The group therapy session afterwards had gone particularly badly, with the facilitator starting a row about politics. This was unprofessional and she later apologised, but not before I had stopped trusting that the room I was walking into was going to feel safe enough for me to start talking about various hideous things from my past.

It's not particularly surprising that I ended up connecting my ride with Penny to the therapy session. Despite being pony-mad as a child (I lived in Surrey: I played the flute, rode ponies and learned ballet, as was apparently compulsory for all good girls in Surrey at the time), I had never really stopped to consider quite how big the trust between rider and horse normally is. We trust an animal far more powerful and heavy than us to carry our bodies on its back. The animal trusts us enough to let us clamber aboard, to direct it and to look after it. Horses have the means to stop that relationship at any time. Mostly, they don't.

I had experienced what happens when that relationship of trust breaks down, and it was, well, traumatic. Most PTSD sufferers struggle to trust anyone, and I've written earlier in this book about how little I trusted my partner, friends, colleagues and family to do anything that was in my interests. My imagination did enough hard work in creating scenarios in which I couldn't trust people. When my trust was really broken, it was devastating.

Even though I knew full well that horses threw people from time to time, and even though I'd felt the rush and thud of coming off before, I'm not sure I would have gone back to Holly Lodge had it not been for Andreas Liefooghe. He runs the centre, which offers 'horse sharing' packages to the public. Those sharing packages fund the real work of the centre, known as Operation Centaur, which is equine-assisted psychotherapy for people with addictions, and children in the care system. Andreas is a psychotherapist himself. I'd mentioned in passing to him that I was riding because it helped my mental illness. Perhaps he remembered that, or perhaps he was just wondering why I'd missed three weeks at the stables. Either way, he dropped me an email one day, asking if I wanted to try riding out with just him and Penny.

When I arrived, Penny was unwittingly offering an explanation for her bad behaviour of a few weeks before. She was busy shoving her bottom into the face of one of the male horses. This, for the unacquainted, is what passes for a pick-up line in the equine world, which again makes our own undignified human rituals seem a little better by comparison.

Normally when we're in the park, we trot and canter as well as bumble around at a walk. But that day, we only walked the horses. We went off track, and allowed Penny and Andreas' horse Hudson to work out their own way over the uneven ground. Andreas explained that he was letting me work out how to trust Penny again. He also talked to me about how tense I was and how Penny would sense that. To help her calm down, I needed to settle myself, too.

I was privately a bit irritated by this: I'd come riding in the first place to try to calm myself down, and had ended up getting chucked on to the ground. I was also unsure as to how I could calm myself down; as anyone who has been unwise enough to tell an agitated person to calm down knows, this doesn't usually result in someone doing anything other than getting even more irritable. But I didn't want to find myself making contact with the bracken at high speed again, and so I decided that the best way to calm down was to ask Andreas about what Holly Lodge actually did when it claimed to do 'therapy'.

Equine-assisted therapy (EAT) doesn't actually involve any riding. The horse is plodding around next to the walking client, and the session is as much about how the client interacts with the horse as it is about what they want to tell their therapist. Horses, Andreas argued, are deeply empathetic creatures. Not only can they sense when you are nervous as you're riding them, but they can also work out other emotions. I had already spotted this with Penny when her

PMT wasn't raging. I had turned up to ride one day when I was feeling utterly dark. My head was full of angry thoughts swirling like disturbed birds. I'd caught a taxi to the stables as I'd left it so late to get out of the house. Penny had been so gentle with me that day, snuffling into my hands and gently leading me around the park. She knew how much pain I was in. Obviously, she had been somewhat distracted when she started going into season a few weeks later, but I had already experienced what horse empathy can be like, hormones aside.

So horses aren't consistently helpful when it comes to working out how we are feeling. But then the therapy that Holly Lodge does with its clients isn't really about a horse comforting a distressed person. It's not even just about someone learning to trust again. It's also about the things people say when there's a big animal plodding around them.

One of the reasons horses work so well with people struggling with addictions or children in the care system is that these people tend to find it very hard to open up about their feelings. Addictions help them numb their feelings, or the repeated churn of moving from foster family to care home and on again teaches a child that it's not worth building trusting relationships only for them to be broken again. Horses can relax people and act as a distraction that stops the therapy environment from seeming so threatening. They are fascinating creatures and 'people can't stop talking about them when they see them'. They also provoke fascinating responses in clients. Andreas explains:

> Quite often we will have people who say that the horse isn't coming
> over to them 'because it doesn't like me' or 'it's stupid' or 'I'm useless

at this'. And that obviously tells us a lot about where they are because horses don't relate to humans in that way, they're not judgemental. That's the person telling us indirectly how they feel about themselves; that they're worthless and don't deserve to be liked. Then we can work with that.

Operation Centaur at Holly Lodge set out to work with people who didn't already have access to horses, rather than become just another Richmond Park stables for the well-off. And Andreas didn't set out to work with easy clients, either. 'We have always chosen to work with really difficult client groups,' he explained. 'Because I think there is something quite satisfying with being able to at least nudge someone out of the last chance saloon.' One such group of people occupying that saloon is children who are at the very edge of the education system. Expelled from pretty much every school in their area, badly behaved pupils end up in a Pupil Referral Unit (PRU). Often, this is the border between the education and criminal justice systems, with PRU students just a step away from a Young Offenders' Institution. They have complex backgrounds, tough family lives and few people who seem fully on their side by the time they move into a PRU. 'It's like a dustbin of kids that have been rejected, and nobody wants them any more.'

But Operation Centaur does. It takes PRU children into an arena with the shire horses and they are asked to do certain things with the animals, like lead them around a course. Once again, what they say about the horses tells the therapists a great deal about what the children are thinking. But the way the children interact with Andreas and his colleagues is also part of the therapy:

Particularly with the boys, who are fourteen or fifteen years old, they are all just ramming into me like crazy. Every single male figure in their lives is already deeply suspect. But they also want to be able to do what I do because they want these horses to listen to them. They then realise they need to cooperate: all of a sudden there's a motivation for them to work with me.

All they are used to in their lives is constant conflict, but this moves from a conflict model to a cooperative model. We just invite them to come and work with us, and these kids start realising that there is a collegial approach to life. In about five sessions, we can get a group to turn around, and we can go into the PRU and we give them pictures of the horses and reminders of their time there.

'Turning around' for these children is rarely about getting them back into mainstream education as a model student. There are so many factors holding them back, from their family context to the involvement they may already have in the criminal justice system. But Operation Centaur's aim is to 'give them the surprise that they can be successful at something', says Andreas. 'All of a sudden they start doing something right; they are being praised for something because [usually] everyone just tells them how shit they are. We get them to at least experience that there is a different way of being in the world.'

According to Eagala, the umbrella organisation for EAT, horses are being used to treat mental health problems in forty different countries.[9] There are ranches in America working with children and adolescents who are at risk, adults with PTSD, victims of child abuse, eating disorder patients, veterans, and those with anxiety, depression and more. In Saudi Arabia, children and adults take part in EAT to help with anxiety and depression. In Australia, there are centres where the horses help clients with mental health problems, and others where companies can use the animals to help deal with problems in their team. As with assistance dogs, this isn't a surprise in many ways: so many cultures have relied on horses throughout their existence. There's no reason to stop now.

But the evidence base behind this work isn't as strong as it could be. Researchers for the South West Yorkshire Mental Health NHS Foundation Trust and the University of Huddersfield conducted a literature review in 2011 which concluded that 'EAT enhances positive behaviours, reduces negative behaviours and has helped people with mental health problems'.[10] The review added that: 'The studies found indicate that EAT can be as effective as other therapies currently in use and could be an alternative to talking and existing experimental and creative therapies.' But it then called for more comprehensive studies, particularly in the UK. Looking further afield, in Canada, researchers concluded that 'dog and horse-assisted therapy is able to improve mental health function and socialisation in patients with depression, trauma, schizophrenia, and dementia in the short-term, but further research is needed to determine long-term effectiveness and how it compares to standard of care'.[11] A 2014 study of chronic psychiatric inpatients found that those in an EAT group had the largest decrease in violent behaviour out of all the groups (the others were canine therapy, social skills and a control group carrying out routine hospital activities).[12]

In some countries, horses have been particularly helpful in communities where established medical practice just keeps failing.

Australian charity the Telethon Kids Institute found that many of the indigenous children it worked with weren't responding properly to traditional therapy methods. Suicide rates among children and young people in indigenous communities in West Australia are among the highest in the world, and something needed to change. EAT seemed to fill a lot of the gaps left by a counselling room: it mirrored what those working on the programme called an 'Aboriginal world view' of the way people connect with animals and the land. Professor Juli Coffin from the Institute set up a Nguudu Barndimanmanha (which means 'horses making good') in Geraldton.[13] It helped 370 young Aboriginal people with behavioural problems that led to them being excluded from school and developing drug addictions, as well as teaching others leadership skills. The mix of work meant the programme didn't become pigeonholed as something just for mentally ill people, but something that could help everyone. It has now expanded to other parts of the country.

Similarly, those who have taken part in Liefooghe's six-week EAT programme in Richmond Park have all reported increased openness to their own emotions, confidence, the ability to ask for help, trust mindfulness and awareness that actions have consequences.

Not everyone takes quite such a positive view, though. Here's one headline from the *Sun*: 'The shireshank redemption: storm as women lags get horses for "therapy"'.[14] The 2016 story reported that 'prison chiefs have been blasted for sending shire horses into jail to provide "therapy" for hardened lags'. The paper quoted a victims' group calling the Operation Centaur project at HMP Bronzefield a 'disgrace' because it appeared to be making inmates happy, rather than punishing them. But the story also mentioned that a similar project at HMP Portland had seen a 27 per cent reduction in twelve-month reoffending.

The *Sun* is a newspaper I write for and enjoy reading. It often commissions me to write about mental health and domestic abuse, and it has run enlightened and powerful campaigns on both matters. In this instance, it was fairly quoting the response of victims' groups to what appeared to be a rather cushy project involving inmates having fun with some lovely animals. If you're a victim of a crime, you're unlikely to respond particularly warmly to the news that the perpetrator is being given a fun day out with a horse. But if you're someone who doesn't want to see those perpetrators creating more victims with further crimes, then you might be more interested in what actually works to rehabilitate offenders. The problem is that ponies aren't really the first things that come to mind when thinking about therapy or prisoner rehabilitation.

Similarly, when I recorded a Radio 4 programme that included my own experience of riding to combat my illness, I was castigated online by people who said I was presenting an impossibly expensive form of exercise to people who are often too ill to afford it. At the time, I was upset that people couldn't acknowledge that this was my personal story, and that I was merely being honest and open about what had helped me. But in the months since, I've reached a more important conclusion, which is that a potentially significant source of therapy is often written off as a posh frivolity. Oddly, we do not take the same attitude towards the use of horses to help with physical problems: the Riding for the Disabled Association (RDA) tends to be (rightly) universally applauded for the work it does in getting disabled children and adults into the saddle or carriage.

But the RDA cites mental well-being and resilience in its impact assessments of its work, and one of the key things that keeps its riders coming back is the way getting on a horse makes them *feel*. All RDA instructors describe the way a disabled child appears to open up when they are with a horse.[15] We have accepted this happy horsey magic for physical disabilities. It's time to take another look at what these creatures can do for mental health problems, too.

Loneliness

Animals have long been used in care settings to calm patients down: dogs, cats and rabbits are taken on to wards and into nursing homes for therapeutic visits. Stroking a furry creature helps a patient, but these visits are short-lived and so is their impact. What is more powerful is what happens when an animal comes to live with someone who is unwell.

You wouldn't expect a book about dying to be uplifting, but that's the extraordinary achievement of Atul Gawande's *Being Mortal*. It confronts many of the issues around growing old and coming to the end of life that our society would prefer not to talk about, but in a way that makes you want to talk more about them, rather than hide in a corner and cry. One of the loveliest stories the doctor tells as he takes us through what end-of-life care should look like involves two dogs, four cats and over 100 birds. A recently-appointed nursing home physician in upstate New York, Bill Thomas, was unsettled by the environment he found himself working in. The elderly residents were suffering from what he called Three Plagues: boredom, loneliness and helplessness. And the way to fight these plagues was to bring life into the nursing home, giving each resident a plant, starting a vegetable garden and, most controversially, bringing in animals. Thomas managed to convince his superiors and the state regulators to introduce the animals and birds all at once. It was chaos to begin with, not least because the flock of parakeets arrived before their cages, and had to be shut in a room and then re-caught. One of the dogs defecated on the floor and a nurse refused to clear it up. But Thomas told Gawande what that chaos, that noisy burst of life, had done for the residents:

> People who we had believed weren't able to speak started speaking. People who had been completely withdrawn and nonambulatory started coming to the nurses' station and saying, 'I'll take the dog for a walk.' All the parakeets were adopted and named by the residents. The lights turned back on in people's eyes.

The number of prescriptions per resident fell to half of that of another nursing home nearby. Deaths fell by 15 per cent, which Thomas argued was down to 'the fundamental human need for a reason to live'.[16]

A therapy animal that pops in for half an hour once a week has all its needs taken care of. The patient merely receives it for a little while, before seeing it led down the corridor and away from the ward. But these dogs, cats and parakeets became the responsibility of the care home residents. They gave them a reason to get up and to stay more active than they had previously been.

The same thing happened when a care home in the north-east of England discovered one of its residents was missing the hens he had kept before entering the home. The charity Equal Arts decided to buy a second-hand hen house and six hens. That started the HenPower project, which has spread across the region and is now opening up in other parts of England. The reason for its success is that care home residents are expected to look after the hens, rather than just petting them every so often.

The volunteers, or Hensioners as the programme calls them, designed the hen houses and runs, and took over the day-to-day care of the creatures. They then found that other people in the community were fascinated by the hens, which meant they started to build relationships with them as they explained hen-keeping. They took the hens into local schools, held competitions to name each bird, made hen-themed cards and even started breeding more. As with Thomas' menagerie of parakeets, cats and dogs, the hens led to a reduction in the need for antipsychotic medication, lower levels of loneliness and reduced depression.[17]

Hens demand attention as soon as the light breaks. When I kept four chickens in my back garden, I would hear them clucking and calling from 4.45 a.m. in midsummer. I bought my neighbours off with regular deliveries of their fresh, rich yellow-yolked eggs. They are not demanding creatures to care for: you need to make sure they have adequate feed and water, collect their eggs every day and muck out their coop once a week. Those chores do not take up oceans of time or great reserves of energy, but just watching the birds go about their routines as you go about looking after them is incredibly satisfying, too. They form complex social hierarchies, with one hen often becoming a dominant, rather bullying character, and chasing less high-profile birds out of the way. They enjoy dust-bathing to clean their feathers. Watching a dust bath is one of life's great pleasures. The chickens peck and scratch out craters in the ground, before flinging their bodies into the holes and pecking more dirt loose. Then they huffle their feathers, roll, twist and thud their legs to loosen the soil. The birds often do this in pairs, huffle-thudding around one another in the bird equivalent of a Jacuzzi.

Some breeds of hens are known for being particularly sociable: warrens, which are the common brown colour and very good egg-layers, also enjoy spending time with humans. My warren hen, Rosie, would happily follow me around my garden, 'helping' me with tasks such as weeding and destroying slugs. She loved nothing more than finding a coven of slimy slugs and slurping each one of them down happily. When I brought the girls a bucket of porridge on cold mornings, they would run excitedly towards me, their bodies tilting from side to side like little triangles.

Keeping my birds well-fed and safe gave me a reason to get up every morning, but I was a healthy young woman who needed to get up anyway because a day of work stretched ahead. Elderly people in homes don't always have that same compulsion to do something with their day. They can deteriorate mentally and physically, not because their age and illnesses make that inevitable, but because they have no reason to exercise their bodies and minds. Loneliness is a great plague in the West and was a problem that caught the heart of British Labour MP Jo Cox, who promised when she was elected to Parliament to tackle the epidemic in her constituency.

Cox was murdered in June 2016, and her family and friends vowed to continue that mission, setting up the Jo Cox Commission on Loneliness. It examined the devastating impact of loneliness, not just on elderly people, but on the whole population. The statistics it collated were miserable: over 9 million British adults are often or always lonely, 50 per cent of disabled people will be lonely on any given day and for 3.6 million people aged sixty-five, TV is the main form of company. Three out of four GPs say they see between one and five people who are mainly in their surgeries because of isolation, and it costs UK employers £2.5 billion a year. The Commission cited one rather contested claim that 'weak social connection is as harmful to health as smoking fifteen cigarettes a day'.[18] That comparison might be unhelpful, but it remains the case that loneliness does damage health. It can be both a consequence and an aggravator of mental health problems.

Animals can be much better companions in themselves than the TV, but they also increase the number of social interactions a lonely person has. If you walk your dog, you bump into other dog owners and end up chatting about your daft pooches. Friendships form over years of waiting for the dog to finish his business. The chicken keepers found other members of the community were fascinated by their feathered friends. Their visits to schools and the need to work together to solve hen-related problems improved their social bonds. And all this from animals that cannot even talk.

HenPower was never intended to be a project where birds are whisked in and out of an old person's bedroom. If nothing else, it is nigh-on impossible to catch a hen when you really need to, and so the whisking would be of a very frenzied, chaotic sort. I know this only too well, having tried to catch one of my birds one morning when in a hurry to get to work. I ended up skidding in the mud, sliding down a hill and bringing the fence down on top of me, all while wearing my smart work clothes, which I'd stupidly already put on to 'save time'. Not a good plan. As a result, the organisers of the HenPower project argue that we shouldn't expect therapy animals to have a significant long-term impact on someone if they just visit irregularly.

This raises important questions about what really counts as a 'therapy animal' and what doesn't. Sure, contact with animals tends to lift most people, but is that sufficient to be considered 'therapeutic'? Andreas Liefooghe worries that not enough care is being taken around the use of the word 'therapy', with well-meaning but unqualified animal owners trying to offer something they shouldn't:

> We need to have a debate over the word 'therapy'. Just because you have a therapeutic experience, doesn't necessarily make something therapy. There are quite a lot of riding schools and even the British Horse Society is promoting the idea of riding as therapy. We need to be very, very careful with that. It's all good if everything goes well, but what if people start doing armchair psychotherapy with people when they haven't actually got the training to put things back in order? Or they'll start burning out because they don't know the important things to do around your own mental hygiene. This is a skilled job, to therapeutically work with someone. We need to make sure it is being done safely.

The Emotional Support Squirrel

Before reading this chapter, you might have been more aware of the weird side of 'therapy animals'. They've been getting a lot of press recently, and not for particularly positive reasons. In 2018, an 'emotional support squirrel' was booted off an internal flight in Orlando, America, because it contravened Frontier Airlines' ban on rodents in the aircraft cabin.[19] Had the passenger brought an emotional support dog, cat or even *miniature horse* on board instead, this would have been absolutely fine, but squirrels were a definite no. There have been emotional support turkeys, kangaroos, alligators and one recorded attempt at boarding an emotional support peacock, though the bird was banned from a United Airlines flight because it was too big, even without its tail in full display.[20]

I must confess that when I came across the emotional support kangaroo, peering in bewilderment at its mile-high surroundings, I laughed so badly that my dog thought I was in pain and started pawing me to try to help. He is proof that animals *can* provide emotional support, and the reason some airlines allow their cabins to resemble petting zoos is that some passengers say their fear of flying is so great it can only be overcome by the calming presence of an animal. We know from this chapter that their assertions have some grounding, but the problem with 'emotional support animals' is that they are often confused with the assistance and therapy animals trained by professionals. It is impossible to train a peacock to behave in the way a registered assistance dog can: there is no animal whisperer on earth who can teach the bird to defecate only when its harness is removed, for instance.

In the States, you merely need to go online and spend around $80 on a certificate stating that your kangaroo is an emotional support animal, and hey, presto! This takes no account of whether the animal is trained or even safe around others. By contrast, genuine assistance dogs take a couple of years to train and have their suitability tested before they are given the legal protections which allow their owners to take them into shops and other areas where pet dogs are banned. Not all prospective assistance dogs pass the test because of this: they might make lovely pets, but if they can't behave in the very restrained way required of them, then they won't be able to assist their owner. Emotional support animals don't have the same levels of access as service animals, but they do get the chance to fly in an aircraft cabin rather than the hold, and circumvent landlords' bans on pets in a home too.

What this leads to is those with properly trained dogs being mocked or even prevented from using them in the way they should be entitled to. Organisations stop believing that any animal can be trusted to behave properly and not defecate all over the place or attack other passengers and visitors. There is also the possibility that emotional support animals become a way of owners actively avoiding proper therapy and treatment: dogs are wonderful companions and can, as I've explained, make life feel a lot more bearable, but even when it comes to the veterans using them to help manage their PTSD, their effect comes partly from the CBT offered to the owners as part of their training. A pet can be a huge help, but not if it's attacking people around it or making life harder for someone who really needs a properly-trained service dog to be able to leave the house.

It also isn't particularly fair on an animal if it becomes the focus of an owner's internal pain without proper professional support – or indeed if the animal itself has a fear of flying. Wouldn't an emotional support miniature horse then deserve its own emotional support squirrel? Why not just cordon off a section of every aircraft for an emotional support petting zoo?

The horses at Operation Centaur help people confront the problems their mental illnesses are trying to keep locked tightly away. Veterans with Dogs teaches its owners to listen to their animals so that they can live as safe and full a life as possible. Hens help elderly people feel part of a community. Pets undoubtedly have their place too, but as with many treatments prescribed to people with mental health problems, it's worth being honest about how far your pet bird can really take you. The beautiful patterns in a peacock's tail are mesmerising, but they cannot change your own destructive thought patterns for good.

CHAPTER EIGHT

———

Does It Really Work?

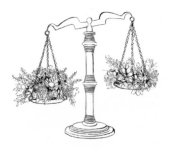

How much can the great outdoors really help you? It's here that I should strike a rather, well, depressing note. It can't cure you. To underline this, flick back through the pages of this book and note how many of the case studies involve patients making a complete recovery. In fact, some of the people I interviewed about their swimming, naturalism and running have had serious mental health crises since we spoke, with a number even being hospitalised.

So does this mean that the great outdoors is just another form of the quackery that I criticised in the first chapter? No, but it's worth setting the Natural Health Service in its proper context so that it can really help, rather than hinder, people who are sick. The people who I mentioned above who have had hospital visits are not examples of a failure of the great outdoors or of their own efforts to manage their mental illnesses. They are an illustration of just how pernicious psychiatric problems can be. You take the pills, you go to therapy, you watch the birds, run the marathons and dive into the cold lakes, and still that utter monster manages to sneak its tentacles around your mind once again. Yes, looking after yourself might help you manage the symptoms day-to-day and may even reduce the likelihood of a serious relapse. But just as flupentixol doesn't promise that a sufferer of schizophrenia will never again believe that the floor is actually boiling water, so the care offered by the great outdoors isn't a guarantee of a healed mind.

Some illnesses come and go; others are cyclical and last a lifetime. Each illness, each person, each situation, will need a different regime of treatment, occupational health and different doses of the great outdoors. Each stage of an illness will require something different too. But while that something might well help someone to live with their illness or experience much less severe symptoms, it still might fail to cure someone.

I know this full well myself. Despite trying every activity that I've detailed in the preceding chapters, I'm still sick as I finish this book. I am still on a high dose of sertraline and still need psychotherapy. I still have days when I either cannot get up to go into work or when I need to leave work suddenly, my face folded into what I hope will be an expression of such concentration that no one will try to stop me for a friendly chat as I walk out. I took many months longer than promised to finish *The Natural Health Service*, not because I am a lazy journalist who pushes deadlines as far as I can (though most editors will verify that I have a compulsive habit of filing fifteen minutes after whatever deadline they set, no matter how tight or generous), but because of the amount of time I spent off sick, unable to write a thing. I can gain great repose from a wood and its trees, but these do not stop me from seeing the things that trigger flashbacks. I can manage those flashbacks so much better thanks to cold-water swimming, but that still doesn't stop me from having days when my madness manages to glue my limbs to the mattress, and I end up congratulating myself not on swimming an extra length in icy water, but on managing to get up and clean my teeth before disappearing back to bed.

At an early stage in my recovery, I would talk about my efforts to 'beat' depression. Mental health culture applauds that, too: celebrities talk about their battle with depression in the past perfect tense when for most of us it is an ongoing struggle. It is not so much a war fought on a battlefield with triumphant noises and medals but an ungainly slip-slide up a muddy hill. I have now realised that I may never entirely close up the black hole inside me. My best hope is that I study it as well as a walker attempting Helvellyn might, knowing its crags and drops well enough that I stand a better chance of not falling into the darkness too often. This is not a dispiriting thought: in fact, it has come as a relief, as it means I am not constantly yearning for the days when I am better again. Instead, I know that it is better to learn to love what it is that I can enjoy right now, sane or not.

Some of my best adventures have occurred when I have not been very sane at all. When I am too ill to work, I take myself off on my bike or out for a walk, and the things I have found while exploring are so memorable as to make me feel that, at the very least, I am not wasting the life I have ended up with. Yes, I would love to have surged ahead further in the political world – there have been weeks when I have been bursting with pride that I managed to work four full days while my contemporaries have been taking promotions, signing new contracts and generally glittering – but I haven't lost everything.

That's not to say that I see my mental illness as a blessing in disguise. An odd compliment that some people have thrown to me is that you cannot be successful without being a bit mad. I know what they are trying to say, pointing to all the artists, authors and other brilliant people who have struggled with mental illness of one kind or another. But I'm afraid I do not believe this to be true. PTSD has stolen a great deal from me. It also came along after I had established myself in my dream career. I know that it has made me a more empathetic journalist, that it has helped me understand better the chasm between the warm words of politicians and the reality of healthcare for a patient. But it cannot be that this illness has made me who I am when its effects have all too often been to prevent me from even being able to read and understand a newspaper.

Another well-meaning thing people say to those who are struggling with mental illness is 'Have you tried X or Y?' It's a common response, often from those who are desperate to help fix the problem that their friend has brought to them, when mental illness can't just be fixed like a dodgy computer, and generally people tell their friends that they are struggling just because they don't want to feel quite so lonely in the dark moments.

This book is brimming with things that are worth trying to help mental illness. In a number of cases, it has been thanks to friends kindly suggesting that they join me for a swim or try just walking the naughty pony rather than getting nervous that she'll bolt, that I've learned the power of the great outdoors. But it would be a misuse of the Natural Health Service if it becomes yet another thing used – whether inadvertently or otherwise – to make unwell people feel guilty that they're just not trying hard enough. As Wayne Singleton explained in Chapter Five (page 144), not every apparently miraculous exercise works for every person. If you don't enjoy running, it doesn't make you any less committed to trying to look after yourself while mentally ill. Sometimes I am too unwell to face leaving the house and catching a bus to the lido. This doesn't mean I've given up: it just means I'm too sick.

You may have bought this book because you are worried about a friend or family member and want some ideas of how to help them. The best thing is to ask them how best you can support them, rather than bombarding them with a list of things that might help. You may find that they've already tried running and it just didn't do it for them. Or that what they really want is someone to listen to them and agree that, yes, it is unfair that their illness is preventing them from working and enjoying time with family in the way they once did. The best friends I have are the ones who listen and then ask, 'What do you think might help you?'

Panacea or Placebo?

In this book, you have met a lot of people who, like me, believe that their illnesses have at least become manageable or a little less acute as a result of the great outdoors. But the word 'belief' is a difficult one and raises an important question that applies to everything discussed here. How much of the great outdoors is merely a placebo that works because people want it to? Do the people who evangelise via Instagram about Wim Hof's cold-water exploits feel less depressed because everyone told them it would have that effect or because it really has some intrinsic worth of its own?

Most of us know that placebos are an important part of scientific research. We think of them as sugar pills handed out in medical trials where the doctors are trying to work out if a new cancer drug actually works, or prescribed to hypochondriacs who keep bugging their physician with fake illnesses. As it happens, those cancer drugs are now rarely compared with a real placebo because to examine how effective a cancer drug is, you need to give it to a cancer patient, and to give a sugar pill to a cancer patient is quite obviously unethical. It isn't so well known that randomised controlled trials do not use pointless pills as the placebo or that doctors cannot hand out sugar pills with a fake label claiming they are antibiotics, morphine and so on. It's also not particularly well known that the placebo itself *can help you recover from a real illness.*

In his book *Bad Science,* journalist and scientist Ben Goldacre sets out quite how powerful placebos can be. The colour of the pills makes a difference, he explains, with blues and greens more likely to work for depression, while reds and yellows work better as stimulants. Capsules have greater power than tablets, and anything that seems to be a more extreme intervention, like an injection or some kind of machine, has an even greater effect. If a doctor believes in his or her treatment, it is more likely to succeed, and the more time and effort they take with each patient, the more likely that patient is to recover. That's one of the reasons why homeopathy appears to work despite its medicine merely being sugar pills which have been created in a bizarre fashion (a powerful substance is diluted to the extent that it no longer exists and then shaken about against a wooden striking board covered in leather and stuffed with horse hair to resemble a saddle). Nevertheless, homeopaths spend more time talking to their patients than NHS doctors can. Particularly relevant to a book on how outdoor activities can help mental illness is this study, which Goldacre quotes:

> In fact, even the lifestyle gurus get a look in, in the form of an elegant study which examined the effect of simply being told that you are doing something healthy. Eighty-four female room attendants working in various hotels were divided into two groups: one group was told that cleaning hotel rooms is 'good exercise' and 'satisfies the Surgeon General's recommendations for an active lifestyle', along with elaborate explanations of how and why; the 'control' group did not receive this cheering information, and just carried on cleaning hotel rooms. Four weeks later, the 'informed' group perceived themselves to be getting significantly more exercise than before, and showed a significant decrease in weight, body fat, waist-to-hip ratio and body mass index, but amazingly, both groups were still reporting the same amount of activity.[1]

So if you are told that running, or swimming, or gardening has helped a lot of other people, and if your doctor prescribes something because they believe it has helped a lot of people and because the NHS has told them to, then aren't you just receiving a placebo? You'll believe it's going to work. You might need to buy exciting new kit to make it work, like trainers or a wetsuit. Perhaps the extreme nature of the intervention, like swimming in a cold lake or joining a 'Forest Therapy Group', makes it sound like a more powerful treatment and so you put your trust in its ability to help you. Of course you will report feeling better by the end of the session.

I loathed sport at school and can think of very few occasions when two hours on the lacrosse pitch or a session in the pool left me feeling better about the world. Perhaps this was merely down to my attitude: as a teenager, I associated sport with an angry woman in a fluorescent tracksuit bellowing at me, and even angrier lectures at the end of the lesson about how badly wrong I'd got things. It didn't seem that anyone involved in the game really believed it was going to make you happy. But as an adult I started to believe that running could make me happy, that swimming was something that I could do and really enjoy, and that spending two hours at a club training session was something to look forward to. Perhaps the only thing at work here was my new-found belief that sport was good. Perhaps exercise was no more effective than a sugar pill. Or, if it was more effective than that sugar pill, it was only more powerful because it seemed more elaborate, like those fake injections and special machines that Goldacre examines.

One simple retort to this line of thinking is that so long as the activity works, then does it really matter? Given so much of the great outdoors is free, does it really matter if people choose to spend their time outside in the belief that it will help them? If those people benefit from the placebo while also taking their regular medication, then what's the harm?

You could even harness the placebo effect in the way drugs companies do, commissioning research into how their medicines *look* alongside work on whether those medicines actually treat the illnesses they are supposed to. So if a red capsule pill works better as a stimulant than a cool blue tablet, then why not research what forms of exercise people *believe* in more when they are trying to alleviate the symptoms of their mental illness? There might even be ways of segmenting exercise according to different illnesses: do patients with psychotic illnesses respond better to walking, for instance? Why not just embrace the placebo effect and not worry too much about what lies behind it?

There is some merit in this argument, so long as it involves the kind of outdoor exercise that no one can argue with, like going for a nice brisk walk. But what about climbing Mount Everest in your shorts? That's not a risk-free extra therapy, but the sort of thing that could kill you, a bit like throwing away your antipsychotics without talking to your doctor because you think that cold showers might have just the same effect. There are also questions of money with many activities. Should medics be asking you to spend your own limited finances on attending a project which only works because you believe it does? The NHS in the UK is rightly resistant to funding homeopathy, and not just because homeopaths can often tell their 'patients' to ignore conventional proven treatments for heart disease, for instance. Health service chiefs have also concluded that it is wrong to spend money on something that has no clinical evidence proving that it works any better than a placebo. So if the great outdoors is merely a placebo, too, why are many people who normally like to show off their disgust for homeopathy getting so excited about it?

The first thing to consider is that the mind and the body aren't as separate as we like to think. Many of us who argue airily that mental illness is just the same as a physical problem still buy in to the false divide, articulated by the philosopher René Descartes, that the mind and body are made of entirely different substances. We think that something that is given to the body in the form of a pill works without the mind at all, when in fact the mind plays an important part in our perception of and recovery from pain. So while pharmaceutical companies are not without their massive flaws (particularly when it comes to psychiatric research, as it happens), their research on making pills *look* like they'll work better isn't quite as sinister as it seems. If the appearance of a medicine means the mind is able to work better in the recovery process, then why wouldn't you applaud that? Similarly, if you tell someone that a cold swim is going to help their mental health problem, and that means it actually does so more effectively, then why not? It doesn't mean that the activity itself is without value, just that you are ensuring it is going to have the best impact possible. Too often, we write off the power of the mind when it is in fact just as important to our health as our liver.

We also do not fully understand the power of placebo when it comes to mental disorders. While it is well-accepted that placebos can have a real impact on the amount of pain a patient experiences, there is insufficient research into psychiatric placebos. Some critics of antidepressants often cite studies which suggest only negligible differences between the drugs and a placebo for cases of mild depression, but as these studies tend not to include a no-treatment group, it is still hard to say how effective the placebo itself actually is or whether patients are improving regardless of intervention.[2] No-treatment groups are important as they allow researchers to study the improvements in someone's illness that come about just as a result of time and the natural way in which some illnesses can slowly improve. In his book, *Placebo: Mind over Matter in Modern Medicine*, Dylan Evans also points to research suggesting the power of a placebo diminishes if a patient comes to suspect they aren't taking the real drug.[3] So some trials have used 'active placebos', which replicate some of the side effects of antidepressants. This means researchers can test the role that belief has in treating depression. Beyond anxiety and depression, though, there is little work on the placebo effect on mental illnesses such as schizophrenia, whether it comes to drugs or therapeutic activities such as outdoor exercise.

This is why we urgently need more research of a higher quality into mental illness. We need to know how the drugs that treat us work, and how much of a role the placebo plays. We need to know which activities work, and which of those might work best for certain illnesses. Again, we need to better understand the importance of a patient believing that running or gardening will help them. Not only would such research make it easier for people to turn to an activity that could really help them, but it will also weed out the false, poorly-researched claims which can lead a sufferer up the garden path. Understanding the role the placebo effect can play in the Natural Health Service could make it even more powerful.

Do the Drugs Work?

Our society has got so much better at dealing with mental health than the previous generations. We no longer lobotomise patients or lock them up in asylums like Bethlem Royal Hospital that were once open for public entertainment. In the past three or four years, it has become much easier for someone to mention casually that they have depression. But we are still not really taking mental health as seriously as our warm words often suggest.

We are nowhere near reaching the point of what policymakers call 'parity of esteem' between mental and physical health. This is when both sorts of conditions receive the same level of funding and are subject to the same sort of waiting times. Neither are we making the same advances in the treatment of psychiatric problems as we are with many physical illnesses. You'll know someone who has cancer right now, and you will also know someone with a mental illness. But the treatment for the former illness has changed almost beyond recognition within your own lifetime. You'd have to be in the upper years of middle age to be able to say the same about mental health: many of the drugs prescribed today for mental illnesses haven't changed since the 1970s. A few decades ago, many cancers were a diagnosis of death. Today, people can expect to recover from some of those illnesses or live many years in comfort. By contrast, we are only just starting to get an inkling of what might cause some illnesses like depression. The reason for this is that we aren't spending anywhere near enough on research. In the UK, just £8 is spent per person with a mental health condition. That figure is twenty times higher for cancer.[4] This isn't to pitch two horrible illnesses against one another: it would be stunning if we could replicate just some of the advances that cancer has seen, and it's not as if the battle is anywhere near over for cancer, anyway.

There is very little understanding about which drug might work for which patient, something researchers are now starting to work on. My own experience of medication showed that a great deal of treatment for mental illness involves trial and error – and that the errors aren't particularly pleasant.

I was first prescribed an antidepressant which seemed to make me more anxious and paranoid, so the doctor added a second drug which did calm me down, but also made me gain a stone and a half in a month when I'd stayed the same size and weight since I was twenty-one. I wasn't keen to keep swelling like a marrow all the way through my treatment and begged to stop taking it. Eventually we found that a third antidepressant worked better than the others. But it's only been since the dose of that drug, sertraline, was tripled that I've been able to have weeks where I've stayed reasonably sane. This book has been clear throughout that medication is an important part of mental health care. There is nothing more irresponsible than the natural health lobby, which throws away reams of peer-reviewed research and claims that you can cure severe illnesses through diet or hobbies. That's not what this book is about. But it's also fair to say that people with mental illnesses are being short-changed, taking drugs that shorten their lives and make enjoying what time they have harder.

What Makes Good Therapy?

Just as opening your first packet of pills can feel rather daunting, so walking up the path to your first therapy session can be a pretty scary experience. What if you just don't click with your counsellor? Or if they don't think there's anything wrong with you? Beyond all those individual anxieties about meeting someone who is hopefully going to help you untangle the mess in your mind is a wider worry: how do I know if this therapist is any good? The same goes for outdoor activities sold as 'therapeutic'. In Chapter Seven, Andreas Liefooghe at Operation Centaur seemed more concerned about mental safety than he was about the potential for someone being hurt physically while riding one of his horses.

His fears have a wider application than just work with heavy horses. There is a worrying blurring of the lines between therapy and activities which can have therapeutic benefits. Both are extremely valuable, but it's important to understand the difference. Liefooghe is qualified to carry out therapy with clients, and knows how to look after both those unwell people and himself. By contrast, those running 'therapeutic' experiences need to be honest with themselves and others about what's on offer. The act of riding a horse at a local stables may well help a great deal: it made all the difference to me when I was on my first bout of sick leave. But it isn't therapy, and shouldn't be sold as such, not least because someone's fellow riders may have very little understanding of the kinds of illnesses and trauma they might find themselves hearing about. It may not be fair on either the sufferer or the person trying to help them if what is being billed as a 'therapeutic activity' is actually just an activity that might be helpful.

Businesses and charities need to be more honest about what their activities can actually offer to someone who has a mental health problem. And those of us trying to manage our symptoms need to see the division between a swim that helps us privately calm down, and a counselling session with a qualified psychotherapist in a woodland where you are safe to say whatever you need to.

The problem with this is that even the apparently professional world of therapy is very difficult to navigate. There is no statutory regulator of counselling in the United Kingdom, though there are a number of organisations to which therapists can be accredited. But accreditation isn't always a sign of quality. If you're on an NHS waiting list, you might be directed towards the therapy that your doctor feels is most appropriate for your condition, but the waiting list may be years long, or closed altogether. The sessions you are offered could be too limited in number for you to feel you can really trust a therapist – there are things I only felt able to tell my counsellor after two years of weekly sessions – or they could be in a format that you don't feel comfortable with, such as over the phone, online or in person when you'd rather avoid face-to-face contact. If you're looking for a private therapist, you may have no idea what sort of treatment will work best for you or which practitioners are any good. Of course, therapy is so personal that the definition of 'any good' is pretty difficult to pin down, given feeling that you can get along with a therapist is an important foundation to feeling you can tell them about your darkest moments. But there are fundamentals, such as experience, ethics and so on, which are not necessarily guaranteed, even if someone has an accreditation.

In 2019, ITV cancelled the long-running and alarmingly popular programme *The Jeremy Kyle Show*, a modern form of Bedlam in which people with complex social problems and often mental illnesses were exploited for public entertainment. The show stopped running after the suicide of a guest who had taken a lie detector test about his alleged infidelity, even though such tests are widely accepted to be unreliable. It maintained a pretence to look after its troubled guests by sporting a 'Director of Aftercare', who was supposed to set up counselling sessions and so on for people as they left the studio, often with their lives considerably more tattered than when the cameras had started rolling. That Director of Aftercare was Graham Stanier, who was registered as a therapist with the UK Council for Psychotherapy and the Health and Care Professions Council. Another professional organisation, the British Association for Counselling and Psychotherapy (BACP), had previously complained about the way the show operated, suggesting that its 'aftercare' was not in line with the Association's ethical guidelines. Stanier was not a member of the BACP, but his professional practice gave the show a veneer of respectability when in reality it was not sufficiently looking after some very vulnerable people. In a report to the UK's Digital, Culture, Media and Sport Committee, a clinical psychologist and sociology professor claimed that Stanier seemed 'to have little prior knowledge of the participants' backgrounds, often failing to know their names, and in one example the sex of a baby.'

Politicians are confused about how much they want to meddle with the therapy world. MPs have recently been trying – so far without success – to outlaw 'gay conversion therapy', under which homosexual or bisexual people are allegedly taught not to be attracted to people of the same sex. Despite widespread evidence of this practice causing severe mental distress to those who happen to have been born with a same-sex attraction, it remains legal in the UK. Under the coalition government, ministers said there was no need for state regulation of the sector. There might not be: state regulation isn't always the answer. But the current therapy landscape is too difficult for a healthy person to navigate, let alone someone who is desperately sick.

The Jeremy Kyle Show and gay conversion therapy are extreme examples of how poor the oversight of therapists is in this country. But it remains the case that vulnerable people do not know whether the person they might be paying a great deal of money to is really any good, whether in an objective, ethical sense or, more specifically, as someone who can help them. The BACP requires members to have completed an accredited course or pass the organisation's own Certificate of Proficiency. They then commit to terms and conditions which include having a supervisor, insurance, continued professional development and so on, in place. The BACP audits a selection of its members each month to check this. It has a Find a Therapist directory, but, once again, would-be clients don't always know what sort of therapy might work best for them. It's also difficult to measure success in therapy, given how complex some people's problems are. So there's no rating system.

That's just the private world of counselling, though. Public lists for psychological therapies are unbearably long. In Britain, some NHS trusts have had to close their lists entirely, asking patients to try again in a few months' time, as though a mental illness can be paused until the doctor is ready to see you. Even the 'ambitious' targets set by NHS England in its Five Year Forward View do more to reveal the poverty of provision at present: it is considered a big ask that by 2021, 25 per cent of those who need talking therapies will be able to access them.[5] And the Improving Access to Psychological Therapies programme largely applies to counselling and CBT for depression and anxiety, rather than other conditions such as borderline personality disorder, PTSD and so on, which tend to be treated using other, less widespread therapies.

The cost to the NHS of failing to provide these therapies is bad enough: patients left untreated can deteriorate to the extent that they need hospital admission. A psychiatric bed costs around £300 a night.[6] It's not just the NHS that pays for acute mental health crises, though: people who are extremely unwell can often be picked up by the police and, if there isn't a bed, then that sick person can end up in the cells, which is the last place you'd want to be if your head already felt like a chamber of horrors.

Similarly, in America, patients generally wait too long to receive treatment. Mental Health America reported in 2019 that more than half of adults with a mental illness receive no treatment at all.[7] One of the barriers to accessing therapy in the States is lack of insurance, and though the number of Americans who are uninsured is falling, over 5.3 million adults with a mental illness do not have insurance. Even those who do find that their insurer doesn't always step up when they need treatment: their illness may not fall under the company's definition of what is 'medically necessary', or the insurance doesn't cover the cost of the care or therapy needed, which means providers refuse to accept the insurance. Other insurance-based systems, including Germany's, have long waiting lists for mental health therapies, too, which shows that it is not just the British NHS that is struggling to keep up with demand.

Many people may find that aspects of the Natural Health Service keep them going while they wait to see a professional. But just as the emotional support peacocks in Chapter Seven weren't managing to address their owners' underlying problems, so activities in the outdoors that merely maintain someone's condition can't be seen as a substitute for properly regulated and funded therapy.

Routine

All this waxing lyrical about fitting nature into your everyday life is all very well, you say. But what about the winter? What about when it's raining so hard that you feel as though your very bone marrow is soggy? Or when the days are so short that you leave for work in the dark, come home in the dark and can only make out the lumpy outlines of your garden (if you're fortunate enough to have one)?

It's true that a lot of people only notice the great outdoors when the weather is easy. Parks fill up and outdoor swimming venues become crammed with fair-weather adventurers. Likewise, even if you love being outside whatever the weather, that love can subside significantly when your mental health is particularly bad. Or when you are so busy with work, family and other everyday pressures that the outside world has to stay at bay.

So what if you have young children who take up all your waking hours? Or you live in a city and work in a city and everything about your life, from your environment to the state of your mind, seems grey? Is the great outdoors only for those with plenty of leisure time and access to funds?

Look back on the stories in this book. They're more about normal people with normal lives and families and responsibilities than they are about people who seem inexplicably to have the means to float about in a lake every day and still pay their bills. Think of Paul Brook pushing his child's buggy while looking up at the birds above. The city professionals going on Freshwalks or taking a few minutes out of their day to walk around a local park. The city garden. The children in care at Operation Centaur.

As for the weather, what about Kevin Widdowson with his winter twigs? Or my ice swims which taught me to love those mornings when the cold air stings your skin as soon as you lift the duvet? One writer who particularly struggles with winter is Emma Mitchell. She has suffered from seasonal affective disorder for twenty-five years, and her book, *The Wild Remedy*, details the depressive muffling of her mind as the light fades and the temperature drops. She even writes about a journey along the A11 in which she was tempted to act on her suicidal thoughts, calming down as she saw saplings on the central reservation. For her, contact with nature in the winter time is as much of a lifeline as the antidepressants and talking therapy prescribed by her doctor:

> Each year I approach late autumn and winter as though I'm scaling
> a mountain: a seemingly insurmountable peak that looms and can

drain my entire body of vitality. The foothills can be daunting and I wish I could tunnel through the bloody thing with the giant rock-gnawing drill that carved out the Channel Tunnel. I long to circumvent the months to come and pop up in late February like a five-foot ten-inch mole, just in time to see blackthorn buds swelling. The northern hemisphere has shifted away from the sun and it takes my verve with it. If I succumb to the inexorable downward pull of SAD, it will be almost impossible to free myself from the sofa.

It's in November that each walk I take becomes crucial. Whatever the sky might be doing, ten minutes spent in the wood can alter the balance of the neurotransmitters in my brain that will help shift the tone of my thoughts and work to keep me going. If the sun does emerge, then that dose of mood-shifting brain chemicals is even stronger, and if I spot a jay, some hedge-parsley or a speckled wood butterfly basking on a leaf, then the gentle nature-spotters' high I experience means that the walk is even more medicinal and I can return home feeling almost ebullient, in defiance of the approaching winter.[8]

The more we observe nature, the more we realise how creative it is at finding a way to survive, even in the worst of conditions. Plants have learned how to grow all over the world. Trees look after one another, but they can only get so far up a mountain before they dwindle away. Grass, on the other hand, has worked out how to grow almost anywhere. There are fish that can deal not just with the darkness of the deep ocean, but also the pressure that can crush metal.

We are part of nature and we have evolved with nature to cope with and thrive in our circumstances – whatever they might be. All of us can find a way of surviving in whatever niche we end up in. Many of us might need help with this, which is why social prescribing is so important. Mental health workers who have the time to sit with a patient and understand not just their illness but also their interests can save lives and money. They can work out that spending an hour every day travelling to and from a lake just isn't right for a single mother, but that she might be able to get a friend to look after her children on a Saturday morning in order to do a parkrun. They can understand that an apparently gruff sixty-year-old man doesn't want to sit in a therapy group or indeed go on a special mental health walk, but that he might eventually open up about his feelings of despair while busily coppicing in a local woodland.

While I hope that this book has inspired you, I have deliberately avoided setting out prescriptions and plans for using the Natural Health Service because such rigid guidelines barely work for me from year to year, let alone for everyone else who suffers with the many different illnesses that can hit us. Besides, when people set out their routines, they normally end up appearing like the sort of idealised 'day in the life' articles that end up going viral on social media; those stories from apparently very successful executives who claim to rise at 5 a.m. for an hour of yoga and who only ever eat salad leaves and something called activated charcoal. It's impossible to imagine anyone normal having even one day in the whole of their life that really complies with these alleged regimes. Life is messy, often gloriously so. Rigid plans tend to lead to disappointment and self-flagellation.

But what if you do try to organise your weeks around certain important Natural Health Service treatments? I have learned the hard way that failing to prioritise outdoor exercise when I'm busy means firstly that I don't do that exercise, and secondly that I tend to struggle mentally as a result. Now, I work out when I can swim and run each week, and protect those times fiercely, even if it means turning down extra work. It's an easy trade-off, when I know that looking after myself keeps me well enough to work every day, rather than pushing myself for a few days before collapsing. Even at political party conferences, which are famously busy and unhealthy times of year for those in my world, I make sure I'm going for runs or short walks outside. I can't afford not to.

It's also important that the people around you understand why you need this time outdoors. I have spoken very publicly about my mental illness, partly because I thought I might be able to help a few other people, and partly because it would better explain my mysterious absences, cancellations and erratic behaviour. But it suited me to speak out. Not everyone wants to be so open, and there is nothing wrong with that. Everyone has differing levels of privacy and openness, and indeed I have kept locked away many things, including the specific cause of my illness and the detail of many of the symptoms. But one thing that makes a huge difference is ensuring that the people who really matter have at least some understanding that you are unwell and of what you need to help you manage your symptoms.

This can be tricky in the workplace, and we will examine what needs to change about this in the next chapter. But in the UK and many other countries, employers do have a duty to make reasonable adjustments for their staff, and it may well be that your HR department can help you get, for instance, a little protected time at lunch so you can go for a walk outside, starting later and finishing later if that means you can better cope with the side effects of your medication and have a swim or run on the way in.

Your family and friends will be the people most likely to support you through the long haul of your illness. Some people I know with mental health problems say they have a chosen family, rather than the one they were born into, because they are either estranged from their parents or their blood relatives refuse to understand their illness. Others find that their existing friends are wilfully useless when it comes to mental illness, ditching you because they either don't know what to say or because they find it inconvenient that you might need some support, rather than just existing to make them look popular in a bar. But many of the activities in this book will also lead to a new network of friends who could end up helping you stay alive – and who through their own struggles will have a clearer understanding than many of how you are feeling. Loneliness can be crippling, but it is not inevitable.

You Don't Have to Live In a Yurt

People can often be misled into thinking that the great outdoors can only help them if they dramatically change their lives, give up their job and move to a remote bothy. Nature seems so far removed from our normal lives that we set up a false dichotomy. But the stories in this book underline how easy it is to bring the outdoors into any life. You will notice that few of the people who I interviewed have given up work to live off the land, or even allowed their hobbies to become their lives. Jake Tyler is an honourable exception, but his lengthy walk around the United Kingdom helped him work out what his purpose was. Some of those featured in this book gained work as a result of the great outdoors. Others, like me, have managed to stay in their existing careers.

There are many tales out there about how long journeys and challenges have allowed someone to get to know themselves better and reach some kind of epiphany while walking on the road to Dundee. Many of them are so glamorous they have been made into films, like the movie *Wild*, an adaptation of Cheryl Strayed's book, *Wild: A Journey From Lost to Found*.[9] Strayed walked 1100 miles from the Mojave desert to Washington, despite having no prior hiking experience. She dealt with her past and learned about who she was on the way. It's a moving and at times rather harrowing book. Perhaps a more relatable memoir of a big outdoor challenge is *Floating: A Return to Waterlog* by Joe Minihane. Minihane was a struggling freelance journalist in London who developed symptoms of anxiety. Initially, he hid them from his wife and found swimming in the nearby Hampstead Ponds to be a release from his feelings. Having read Roger Deakin's *Waterlog*, Minihane then set himself a challenge to follow in that writer's wake.[10] The project took him much longer than he'd imagined, and became a significant source of anxiety in itself. A cycling accident led to a broken arm which meant he couldn't swim, and he ended up in a counselling room, explaining the mess his head was in to his therapist Mark:

> Over the next fifty minutes, Mark listened as I talked. I told him about how I got het up about small things, felt guilty about taking time off or enjoying myself, and how I'd tried and failed to use swimming as the

panacea for my problems. How I had embarked on my journey on
Roger's trail and how I felt I'd turned it into an exercise in box-ticking,
sometimes losing sight of the joy it was supposed to inspire. I told
him how I tried to keep everything just so and wanted to make things
perfect. How I liked to always be in control. And, most importantly, how
I thought worrying could make that happen.

'You're trying to line your ducks up in a row,' he said. 'And the fact is
that's just not possible. Because life isn't like that. Change is constant
and things happen all the time. Just one thing – swimming, in this
case – isn't going to make you better. Think of life as if you're floating,
bobbing around with all the flotsam. It's essentially a Buddhist theory,
but let's forget the religious aspect. You need to try and see what's
going on around you as largely uncontrollable. In short, you need to
step back and recognise whenever you feel yourself get stressed and
anxious about situations you can't affect, take some deep breaths and
learn to say "fuck it".' 'Fuck it,' I mouthed. 'Learn to say "fuck it".' I grinned
and Mark let out a loud, 'Ha.' Just saying it made me feel better.[11]

In a later session, the pair discussed why Minihane had found that
swimming, the one thing he'd pinned his hopes on to make him feel
better, had become a source of anxiety. He eventually completed his
journey, and concluded that the swims were the start of 'a healing
process, one I knew now would never end'. It's a sensible conclusion
to reach: that even big challenges don't have neat conclusions.

It's also worth noting that people who work with nature full-time
or who are professional sportspeople do not have a magic immunity
to mental illness. Far from it, in fact: many international athletes
have spoken out in recent years about their terrifying experiences

of depression and self-harm, which are often related to their performance on the track or field. The farming community also has an unusually high rate of suicide, partly because of the financial pressures that modern farmers face. Leaving behind your family and immediate community to live on a croft in the Highlands might look appealing, but it does isolate you from the support network you need the most when the chips are down.

Most of us do not have the freedom to set off on a lengthy hike that takes months. Those sorts of stories can transport the reader to all sorts of places, but they can also mislead that nature is something you have to leave your immediate home to experience. And besides, even long hikes come to an end eventually. What is more important is learning to incorporate the great outdoors into your normal life, whatever shape that is.

———

CHAPTER NINE

The Natural Health Service: A Manifesto

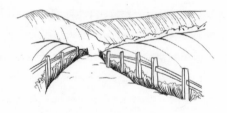

On 5 July 1948, healthcare in Britain changed forever. The National Health Service was launched, promising to meet the needs of everyone, to be free at the point of delivery and to be based on clinical need, not ability to pay. Brits today are so proud of the NHS that we included it in the opening ceremony of the 2012 Olympics, and decorated our windows with 'thank you NHS' posters during the coronavirus pandemic. Politicians – even those who privately think the NHS should be funded rather differently – know that they must praise 'our NHS' and all the people who work in it regularly.

It has been compared to a national religion, albeit the sort that most people are happy to discuss at dinner parties.

Nowadays it is accepted that developed countries should all have some kind of healthcare system. Of course, there's a debate across the world about how involved the government should be in that and the best ways of funding care. But our need for hospitals, doctors, nurses and medicines isn't in doubt. What is less well-recognised is our need for the Natural Health Service.

We have evolved alongside and in nature and so our innate need for it in our lives shouldn't come as a surprise. This book has shown the power of that outdoor-based NHS to help the established health service do its job. It helps seriously ill psychiatric patients calm down and engage better with their therapy. It renews the stressed minds, not just of those who are unwell, but of those who treat them. It fights physical problems which either contribute to or are the consequences of mental illness. It prevents GPs from having to dole out prescriptions for years or repeatedly see patients who need a social network, not a doctor. It helps children let off steam, rather than allow it to build up and fester into something diagnosable and lifelong. It saves lives.

Much of the great outdoors is free at the point of access. We do not pay to walk down the street to our local park or to watch birds through the window. If you have been given an outdoor prescription by a doctor, you might also be able to fund equipment that you cannot otherwise afford in order to enjoy the great outdoors even more.

This NHS is not a behemoth organisation so confusing that few within it can really map its different structures. It is a loose network of charities, individuals, homes, gardens and local authorities which can, despite a lack of official branding or national debate, save lives.

But while the British National Health Service is oversubscribed and struggling to balance its books, the Natural Health Service's waiting rooms are often empty. Too few of us see nature as essential to our lives, whether we are healthy or in need of a spell on a ward. Too few of us realise that it can form an important part of our therapy when we are unwell – or seriously enhance our well-being if we are not. We don't see the right to green spaces as being fundamental in the same way as we do proximity to a good emergency department. Many of us erect artificial barriers to getting into the great outdoors. We presume that nature is a place we need to travel to, that it's expensive and – as proof of our disconnect with it – that it can be threatening, dirty or dangerous. We view time outdoors as a luxury to save for holidays, not integrate into our working days in the same way as we find time to have lunch or pop to the shops. This is absurd: we are part of nature and we need nature.

We need to change our view of the great outdoors. It cannot stay as a luxury. It has to become something that individuals, businesses, governments and societies see as being a right: something so essential that any threat to it is debated as hotly as the closure of a local hospital.

This mindset shift must include those working within the formal medical sphere: doctors and other healthcare professionals are often so wedded to a biomedical model that they struggle to see how important horticultural therapy might be in someone's recovery. When I met Peter O'Hare at Bethlem Royal Hospital, he rather tactfully suggested that the one thing he'd really like to change would be for doctors to realise that the outdoor occupational therapy that his team runs isn't an optional extra while someone is an inpatient, but an integral part of their treatment, helping them recover as much as their drugs and their therapy.

Britain's National Health Service is so popular that it features in every single political party manifesto at every single election. It would be unimaginable for it not to. The great outdoors enjoys the odd platitude and promise to protect the environment, but rarely with an acknowledgement that to do so would also be to better protect our health, as well as the flora and fauna within it.

What would a manifesto for the Natural Health Service look like? It would need to set out the value of the great outdoors in helping our minds, both in terms of the improved outcomes for patients and the money this service can save the public purse and wider economy. It would promise a shift in the way that politicians see the great outdoors from being something pretty to something that everyone must be able to enjoy as part of their everyday lives. It would also promise a shift in wider society, with parents, teachers, charities and healthcare professionals turning to the great outdoors as an essential part of staying healthy, and getting better. And it would promise to address the many barriers obstructing this change from happening.

An Unhealthy Service

The most obvious obstruction is the way many health services treat mental illness. While I have spoken to many doctors, nurses and others working in the NHS who believe passionately in the importance of the great outdoors, it would be remiss of me not to report what all of them have said about what's undermining it. There has not been a single interview that I have conducted – with clinicians or sufferers – that hasn't featured someone pointing out the inadequacy of mental health care in the UK. In fact, for so many people it is the case that the second worst thing after what their illness does to their mind is what the NHS cannot offer them by way of treatment. The same goes for other developed countries too: even those with the sort of healthcare systems that policymakers love to praise still have a gap between their mental and physical provision.

The 2010 coalition government committed to parity of esteem between the treatment of mental and physical health. But this is nowhere near being realised yet, at any level. It's not just the waiting lists for the most common therapies or the lack of access to some of the more complex treatments. It's not just the waiting list for an outpatient appointment with an NHS psychiatrist either (if you're able to get on that list at all) or the dearth of beds on inpatient wards. It's also the fact that 'crisis care' services are often only open between 9 a.m. and 5 p.m., as though mental illnesses only deteriorate during working hours. Worse than that, it's the way politicians today seem to think they are doing a good job if they merely talk about mental health, offering sugary words about lifting the stigma, yet never managing to stump up the really big sums of cash needed to help people who, stigma or not, are getting sicker because they are not receiving the right treatment.

Now the temptation among politicians might be to produce equally lightweight words about the value of social prescribing, as if done badly it doesn't involve the kind of outlays of cash that NHS treatment and therapy do, or indeed the amount of money necessary for improving the drugs on offer. Some social prescriptions may keep some patients from ever needing a higher level of mental health care, but many will still require therapy, and they will get sicker if they are left to languish. So any minister worth his or her salt cannot focus on one aspect of care while ignoring the others.

In Chapter Four, we met Jacob Krzanowski, sustainability scholar at the Royal College of Psychiatrists. While he believes mental health inpatients can benefit a great deal from walking groups, he also worries that staff are stretched so thinly that they cannot offer the kind of support that patients need, let alone taking on a new commitment:

> Under the state of austerity in this country and its compounded impact
> on mental health, it's easy to seek out the path of least resistance.
> There's so much demand on people's time and attention that there is
> a degree of cynicism on both sides – service users and staff – about
> whether they really have the time to get these projects off the ground in
> a meaningful way.

So as much as the National Health Service can benefit from the Natural Health Service, the latter still needs the former to be healthy in order to work properly. One cannot replace the other.

Do we really know what the Natural Health Service should consist of? While I hope that this book has inspired you about the many different ways in which the great outdoors can help a range of mental illnesses – as well as preventing mental distress from developing into a serious condition – I hope that you have also noticed how many times I have had to couch my assertions about the evidence on offer. There are not yet enough studies to prove which of the many activities in this book really improve which symptoms. We don't know what it is about certain activities that seems to help. This is partly because the really big studies are very expensive, and the money for these studies comes from organisations with an interest in spending lots of cash on research, which is generally a pharmaceutical company. There is little incentive for a drugs company to conduct research into an activity which could reduce demand for its products. When the King's Fund examined gardening, it lamented the lack of randomised controlled trials which might provide real evidence for the efficacy of horticulture-based interventions. In some cases, a strong placebo effect may well be in operation. In others, we just don't know which illnesses will respond particularly well to a certain activity.

I could quite easily have replaced the word 'activity' here with medication or therapy. We do not even know why antidepressants work in the way that they do. We do not know if they are the best kind of treatment for depression, let alone how to match the different types of antidepressant on offer to different conditions. The same goes for antipsychotic medication. And while the side effects of the great outdoors include muddy clothes, aching legs and sometimes overly cold feet, the side effects of psychiatric medicines are of a whole different order. These drugs are old and clunky, and there is not nearly enough research going into improving them.

In the previous chapter, we touched on the power of the placebo effect. I have been painfully aware as I have written up the often scant evidence backing up the various interventions in this book that I have used many more words to describe people's individual experiences. Some psychiatrists have insisted to me that there is nothing wrong with that: anecdote is not the singular of data, but neither is it useless. But then again, the proponents of homeopathy often say, 'Well, even if there isn't much scientific evidence yet, all I can say is it worked for me.' In the case of homeopathy, of course, there is a fair body of scientific evidence that it *doesn't* work, and so that 'yet' is somewhat redundant. The NHS describes the principles of homeopathy as being 'scientifically implausible', and in 2017 recommended that GPs and other doctors should stop prescribing it.[1] But are we at risk of creating a new homeopathy in the form of social prescribing? Am I merely a slightly more plausible-sounding version of a homeopath, preaching to my friends that 'All I can say is that jumping into a partially-iced lake has really helped me'?

We often do not know how good the therapists offering outdoor-based or animal-assisted interventions actually are. In some cases, they may be deeply unethical or simply poor quality. Politicians have been wary of overarching regulation of the counselling sector, but there is such variability and so much complexity in which organisation really represents good-quality therapists that patients definitely deserve better than the tangled landscape that currently exists. Many therapists don't have enough of a statistical evidence base to know if what they're doing really works or if it's just based on anecdotes of coincidences and patients recovering as they would given time.

There is certainly some serious research suggesting that the great outdoors as a mental health treatment really works. But, more broadly, we really need more serious investigation into how we treat mental illness that includes drugs, therapy and activity.

The mental health research charity MQ wants to change this. Its founders were so dispirited by the disparity between advances in the treatment of physical illnesses and the tiny gains made when it came to mental health problems that they set up the first major charity funding scientific research into mental illness. Its projects include working out how to match treatments to patients, rather than just leaving doctors to experiment with a range of different medicines; increasing life expectancy in schizophrenia; trying to understand the relationship between serotonin and depression; and preventing repeated suicide attempts. As a charity, it wants people to fundraise for it in the same way that cancer charities see thousands of sufferers, their friends and relatives don fundraising vests every year. But it also campaigns for the government to release more funding for mental health – and for pharmaceutical companies to do the same. 'Big Pharma' has a bad name in today's society – and not without reason – but its money has also been behind many research breakthroughs in the treatment of deadly illnesses such as cancer. Now is the time for this success to visit mental health.

Fighting the Stigma

There are, of course, many reasons to be hopeful that we will see the same research and funding success in psychiatry as we have in oncology. The way we talk about mental health has changed beyond recognition in the past decade. It started with pioneers, who chose to face down the brutal stigma attached to mental illness and talk openly about their own afflictions. Sportspeople have been instrumental in this. From the way the *Sun* changed its coverage of Frank Bruno's psychiatric problems after a public backlash, to the personal stories told by elite cricketer Marcus Trescothick, Dame Kelly Holmes and a host of footballers, there is now recognition that some of the physically strongest people in our society can nevertheless find themselves mentally ill. Celebrity culture has almost reached saturation point when it comes to talking about mental health, but perhaps with less of a profound impact: for every Carrie Fisher or Stephen Fry who refused to shy away from the grinding reality of illness, there's another star who ends up making depression seem like just another thing to be 'beaten', preferably with a slightly bizarre diet or expensive lifestyle choice.

Former New Labour spin doctor Alastair Campbell is one person who helped shake up the political world's aversion to mental illness. In 2012, a group of MPs used a backbench debate in the House of Commons to talk about their mental health problems. It was the first time parliamentarians had done this, and it had a profound effect. A couple of years later, I was sitting in a pre-speech briefing from Nick Clegg's spin doctors about what he was going to say to the Liberal Democrat conference the next day. He had decided to focus on mental health, the aides told us, and he wanted to make it as easy to talk about depression at the school gate as any other subject. As soon as the adviser had said this, a journalist sitting behind me in the windowless basement room of the Glasgow conference centre snorted with derision. 'I mean, that's just not going to happen, is it?' he muttered to one of his colleagues. 'People aren't going to start talking about their depression in public.' The journalist in question was a compassionate, thoughtful type. He wasn't mocking mental illness – indeed, he was incredibly kind to me when I fell ill a few years later – but he was quite realistically assessing the chances of what Clegg wanted to happen ever coming true. Indeed, I was struck by the way the Lib Dem leader's advisers managed to tell us that he wanted to break down the stigma while also seeming quite keen to tell us that 'Nick has never had any mental health problems himself'. At that time, in 2014, it did seem rather far-fetched to imagine school mums telling one another that they'd had some time off sick with bipolar disorder. Now, I quite often hear people discussing their depression or general mental health on the bus, in pool changing rooms and in pubs. The stigma is lifting.

The problem is that the stigma isn't really lifting quite as much as it first seems. Though I do find it as easy to overhear mental health conversations when I am in Barrow-in-Furness as I do when I'm in south-west London, it is undoubtedly the case that you'll find it easier to open up about your mental health if you are a white middle-class woman living in the south of England and working in a reasonably secure career. Far less so if you are a man, given that the expectations of 'masculinity' include being mentally 'strong'. A continued stigma around male mental illness is one factor that charities identify in the higher rates of male suicide. Some communities do not recognise mental health problems at all, whether for religious or cultural reasons. Even those who accept they do have an illness still fear the stigma of having counselling, or even fear the therapy itself, given its general portrayal in popular culture.

Worse than that is the pernicious stigma around serious mental illnesses and symptoms which go beyond someone feeling down or seeming overly anxious. Hearing voices? Seeing things? Convinced the government is trying to silence you? The chances are that your symptoms will still attract a degree of fear and ridicule. Even though I have never suffered from psychotic symptoms, I have been dispirited by the disparity between the kind words people offer about my illness and their reaction to my symptoms. On one level, it is entirely understandable that someone would be taken aback by a sudden outburst of anger and a furious volley of messages about how they're apparently plotting against me. On another level, it is quite crushing to know that, two years and several apologies after the incident, that person still looks down on me in a way I cannot imagine they would have if I had vomited on them, for instance.

Society still needs to better understand the reality of mental illness. It does not magically go away as a result of talking openly. It doesn't stop if you have a lot of friends who send you supportive messages, even though those can often take you away from the brink. It is messy, inconvenient, humiliating and life-limiting, and to pretend otherwise does a great disservice to the people trying to deal with a serious diagnosis. Even the relatively well-accepted depression is not merely a deep sadness, but something that can envelop a sufferer in black moods so heavy the person seems rude and can pull everyone else around them down, too. There are many people keen to be kind and encouraging, but few who are really prepared to stick by a friend or partner who is regularly so dark and unresponsive that they too start to feel low.

So we have reached a stage where mental illness is considered acceptable in the abstract, but less so when it comes to the messy reality.

Mental Health at Work

The pernicious stigma is bad enough when you encounter it socially. Far worse when it comes to trying to earn a living. People with mental illnesses struggle to get the same treatment as their colleagues with physical problems. Around 300,000 people with long-term mental health problems lose their jobs each year in the UK, which is double the rate of those without a mental health condition and a much higher rate than physical illnesses.[2] The less common and less well-understood the illness is, the less likely you are to be in work, and this is not wholly down to the debilitating aspects of psychotic conditions, but to employers' reluctance to manage people with such illnesses.

Many conditions can deteriorate, or even develop, as a result of a bad working environment, and employers need to improve the way they approach mental health. Even bosses who don't care much for their staff will see a benefit in ensuring that their workplaces are mentally healthy and that unwell colleagues are properly supported: in 2018, a UK government-backed report estimated that the cost per year to employers of mental health problems is between £33 billion and £42 billion. That report, conducted by chief executive of Mind, Paul Farmer, and Lord Dennis Stevenson, also suggested that the cost to the UK economy as a whole came in at between £74 billion and £99 billion per year.[3]

This review set out six mental health core standards for employers in an attempt to reduce the number of people who end up leaving employment and to prevent mental illness in the first place. These are:

1. Produce, implement and communicate a mental-health-at-work plan.
2. Develop mental health awareness among employees.
3. Encourage open conversations about mental health and the support available when employees are struggling.
4. Provide employees with good working conditions and ensure they have a healthy work/life balance and opportunities for development.
5. Promote effective people management through line managers and supervisors.
6. Routinely monitor employee mental health and well-being.

The way we are working is changing as a result of coronavirus. Lockdown meant even the most committed office creatures suddenly started to see the benefits of working from home at least a few days a week. It gave them more time to exercise and to see family (for those with young children, of course, lockdown meant the unenviable opportunity to work while also stopping a toddler who had no childcare from trashing the house). Now there is a chance for us to reshape work more widely so that it actually works for our minds, rather than continuing along traditional lines for the simple reason that this is the way things have always been done. Much of this work is out of the scope of this book, but then again, there are many ways in which employers can use the great outdoors inside their workplaces. The research we encountered in Chapter Two about the value of natural views in improving mental well-being (page 5) is clearly pertinent here, for instance. Providing employees with good working conditions might mean a company ensures they are getting a chance to see natural light, to go outdoors into a pleasant area – rather than by a bin store – for breaks, and that there are plants in the office (and plants that people look after, rather than dead plants that make the whole place seem even worse). A healthy work/life balance isn't just about discouraging presenteeism, whereby someone turns up to work even though they are manifestly too unwell to perform their role.

It's not even just about line managers refraining from bombarding their staff with emails late at night to the extent that no one ever really switches off from the working day. It's also about a workplace culture where people are actively encouraged to look after their mental and physical health. Office running clubs, volunteering opportunities in the great outdoors, and even meetings held while going for a walk around the nearby park don't really require that much of an organisational change. My own editor often suggests that we walk around St James's Park when having a meeting, rather than staying cooped up indoors. It's good exercise and I'm certain that we cover a great deal more than we would in a more sterile environment. When Michael Di Paola described the atmosphere on his Freshwalks to me, he compared it to the 'sort of people who would come along to a piss-up in the pub'. There's nothing wrong with spending time with your colleagues in the pub. But does it have to be the only way in which work teams socialise? Could a walk actually help to bond you far more than a piss-up? It would also do more for your employees' mental health than a session in the pub. And it might avoid some of the awkward moments that happen at the end of the work drinking session.

Bosses can take inspiration from the way in which sporting organisations such as England Athletics have set up a network of mental health ambassadors in running clubs. Mental health is no more the primary aim of an athletics club than it is a commercial organisation, but both have good reason to take a strong interest in it. Just as there are qualified first aiders in offices, so there could be qualified mental health first aiders, who are also known to all employees as someone they can turn to if they're struggling. Those mental health workers can also ensure that the workplace is the kind of environment that encourages matter-of-fact conversations about mental health. This isn't about making everyone hug one another at the start of the day, or that everyone's private business is discussed in the office. It's more about ensuring that mental illness isn't mocked as a sign of weakness, but dealt with in the same tone as a physical ailment would be. In unionised lines of work, trade union representatives might take this on as one of their responsibilities.

Individuals can make their own changes, too. I rarely catch the Underground into my office now, preferring instead to cycle. It means that by the end of the day, I've spent nearly two hours outside and active. I see so much on my bike: an owl swooshing across the path in a local wooded area, wild flowers coming and going on the verges, and plane tree leaves squashed into a screen print against the tarmac. Of course, it helps that when I arrive at work, I have the most secure cycle parking in the world: there's something about all those police with machine guns milling around the Parliamentary Estate that deters a would-be bike thief. Other organisations can help with cycle-to-work schemes and secure bike racks.

My desk in the House of Commons exists in a strange twilight world, as the blinds on the large mullioned windows are often drawn to prevent the sunlight blinding my colleagues. When I returned to work, I decided that the piles of old House of Commons order papers and reports from obscure all-party parliamentary groups that I'd never read might not be hugely conducive to keeping me calm when I was still sufficiently unwell as to feel on edge the whole time. I was also aware that my mind couldn't take long periods of concentration without becoming severely fatigued, which tended to lead to mad paranoia or outbursts of anger towards perfectly innocent colleagues. So one morning, I turned up early and cleared the desk of many years' worth of mess. I found a few things under the piles that I thought I'd lost, then recycled the rest. I stuck photos of some of my favourite Cumbrian views on to the small screen behind the desk and brought in four or five shade-tolerant houseplants to make my working environment just a little more soothing.

This didn't make my return to work a blissful slide back into my old way of life. Far from it. I started back in December 2016, but ended up going off sick again in April 2017, returning only in the autumn of that year. It took another year and a half before I really settled into a new normal pattern of working. But improving my immediate working environment did improve my mental comfort just a little. I could stare at the Fibonacci pattern made by the spines on my cactus or at the view of Ullswater in the autumn, and feel at least a little more removed from whatever was muffling my head so badly. It was a marginal gain of the order that a professional cyclist makes when he starts shaving his legs, rather than a vast improvement.

Similarly, the twenty-minute break I took in the middle of each day to walk outside also helped keep me on an even keel just a little. I would walk out of the Parliamentary Estate and into the nearby Victoria Tower Gardens or St James's Park, turn my phone off and get my short nature fix. This did reset me a little, giving me more mental energy and calming anxious rumination about whether this colleague hated me or whether I was about to be sacked.

These things were tiny adjustments compared to the efforts that my employer made to keep me in my job. When I was signed off sick, my editor kept in touch with me, suggesting coffees every so often to check how my recovery was progressing and to reassure me that there was no need to rush back. He struck just the right balance between telling me that I was missed and not heaping on the pressure to return to work too early. When I did start to notice that my mind was forming sentences again and that I could face travelling into Westminster, we formulated a plan for my phased return to the office. This involved me working a couple of hours a day for a couple of days a week, and then adding hours as it became clear that I was able to cope. My boss's generosity extended as far as the *Spectator* offering me an extra six weeks' sick leave on full pay, which meant I didn't need to worry about whether I could afford my rent while I was too ill to work. That kindness has been extraordinary and I will never be able to repay it. I am also all too aware that it is out of the ordinary for most employers, and it would be wonderful if other companies learned from the way the *Spectator* has helped me.

Shrinking Nature

Will staff really take up the opportunity of lunch-break walks, plants on desks, outdoor running clubs and so on? As a political journalist, I am very aware that there is a vast gulf between a structure and a culture, with the structures of democracy which provide for the scrutiny of laws often appearing very sound, and the culture of the politicians operating within those structures totally undermining them. This can quite easily be the case in any workplace. Your contract may, for instance, state that you have an hour for lunch each day. But if all your colleagues drop sandwich crumbs into their keyboards while they carry on working, then you're unlikely to think that taking that hour for a walk is acceptable.

Far more pernicious than workplace culture, though, is the disconnect from nature in wider society. We just don't see it as being part of our everyday lives, believing that it only exists in special nature reserves, rather than all around us. Though children have far more status in today's society than they did in previous centuries, they spend far less time outside. Clearly, we do not value nature enough to think it essential that our children come to love it for themselves.

This has a Tinkerbell effect on nature. If we don't notice it or believe that it is important, then we also won't notice or care when it disappears. Take wild-flower meadows. Britain has lost 97 per cent of them since the 1930s, largely as a result of a change in land use following the Second World War. But many of us don't even know what a wild-flower meadow looks like. We presume that those brightly-coloured mixtures of cornflowers, poppies and corn cockles that come in seed packets and are sown by councils in parks constitute wild-flower meadows. Yet these plants are annuals which grow at the margins of arable fields and reseed every year with the harvest and ploughing. In some cases, the flowers in these mixes aren't even native to the UK: the Californian poppy, for instance, is beautiful and common in 'meadow mixes' but the clue is in its name. A real wild-flower meadow will have a rhythm of colours throughout the year and consist largely of perennials. There will be grass, but it won't be so rampant that it chokes out the flowers: semi-parasitic plants like yellow rattle and annual managed grazing will keep the vegetation down. The tapestry of a true meadow is deeper and richer. You might not see all the flowers at once, and you are rewarded for a closer inspection. Fly orchids don't advertise their presence like showy annuals, but are they really worth less for that? Some meadows, of course, knock the breath out of your mouth with far greater force than anything sown from a packet. Marden Meadows in Kent is one such. In early summer, hundreds of thousands of green-winged orchids, *Anacamptis morio*, come into bloom, turning the grass purple. When I rounded the corner one Friday evening and saw these plants for the first time, I let out an involuntary 'Oh!'

The Marden Meadows are protected and owned by the local wildlife trust. But other sites haven't been so lucky. Some aren't technically meadows, but swards along the side of roads, and those frequently fall foul of council or highway authority strimming teams. When I asked plant conservation charity Plantlife why it was that cash-strapped local authorities were spending money on mowing grass verges which were crammed with often rather rare flowers, they replied that this was because councils tend to get complaints from local residents that the area was 'looking messy' and had 'too many weeds'. In the time that I've been writing this book, local complaints have led to the mowing of verges where bee orchids and indeed green-winged orchids grew. Presumably the people who bothered to call up the council to moan about these plants had never stopped to look at their intricate beauty. Presumably they had never got to know what a real British wild-flower meadow looks like.

Those poppies and cornflowers that appear in sown 'pictorial meadows' are still wild flowers, just arable ones. And they're under threat, too, largely from herbicides and the agricultural industry's tendency to destroy the field margins where they flourish. Once again, our lack of understanding about where these plants grow does not help save them: no one notices when they disappear from a cornfield because no one thought they would be there in the first place.

Plants are the start of the food chain, and so chopping them down or digging them up damages everything else that is wild. Yet again, though, we often don't notice. Let's have a look at moths. Most of us tend to notice moths when they have either eaten our clothes or when there's a particularly monstrous one buzzing around the bathroom light. We don't know that they have the most fabulous names, as well as such delicate, classy colourings. There's the angle shades, which has crumpled camouflaged wings resembling an autumn leaf. Or the cinnabar, which is dramatic black-and-red. Almost as dramatic as the Jersey tiger, which has cream and brown tiger stripes and a bright red underwing. The rosy footman is orangey pink with delicate black etchings.

Often, we don't see these details because the moths are dancing in the beam of one light shining into the dark. But nowadays, we're lucky even to see that. In his book *The Moth Snowstorm: Nature and Joy*, environmental journalist Michael McCarthy documents a loss that many of us have barely noticed:

The headlight beams of a speeding car on a muggy summer's night in the countryside, turning the moths into snowflakes and crowding them together the faster you went, in the manner of a telephoto lens, meant that the true startling scale of their numbers was suddenly apparent, not least as they plastered the headlights and the windscreen until driving became impossible, and you had to stop the car to wipe the surfaces clean. (I know there are many other insects active at night as well, but let the moths stand proxy for the rest.) Of all the myriad displays of abundance in the natural world in Britain, the moth snowstorm was the most extraordinary, as it only became perceptible in the age of the internal combustion engine. Yet now, after but a short century of existence, it has gone.[4]

McCarthy found himself covering insect decline a great deal as a journalist, but very few people seemed interested. 'Yet every time I wrote about the snowstorm, people would respond,' he writes. 'They would say how vividly they remembered it, and how now they never saw it…'

Not long after, data arrived to back up the anecdotes that McCarthy had gathered. In 2006, research gathered at agricultural research station Rothamsted in Hertfordshire and published with Butterfly Conservation revealed the moth population to be in freefall:

Of the 337 species examined, two-thirds were declining; 80 species had declined by 70 per cent or more, and 20 of these had gone down by over 90 per cent. In southern Britain, three-quarters of moth species were tumbling in numbers: their total cumulative decline since 1968 was estimated at 44 per cent, while in urban areas, the losses were estimated at 50 per cent. The snowflakes which had made up the snowstorm were simply no longer there.[5]

McCarthy was well-placed to notice their loss, not just as an environmental journalist but as someone who had seen a moth snowstorm for himself. I am much younger and can only just recall small groups of moths dancing in the headlights of my father's car as we drove through rural lanes. Today, when I drive my own car, I see a few moths, generally alone, on Cumbrian roads at night. So I have my own sense of loss, which is that the number of moths I see at night has declined since my own childhood. But I am unaware of the much greater decline that preceded this.

This lowering of expectations between the generations is known as 'shifting baseline syndrome', and it naturally has serious consequences for our natural world. If we are not aware of how much we have already lost, then we come to accept what we have now as normal, rather than an already significantly-altered state. It is not normal that there are no longer moth snowstorms. It is not normal that wild-flower meadows are so rare that people don't have a clue what they look like. Even if we are selfish enough not to care about habitat destruction and species loss, we should worry about ourselves. For in our ignorance, we are making it harder for ourselves to access nature, and thereby making it harder to stay healthy and recover from illness.

Saving Nature

It is still possible, though, for each generation to note the increasing damage being done to the natural environment all the time. We cannot simply expect the Natural Health Service to exist forever if we don't make efforts ourselves to protect it. Climate change, plastic pollution and species loss are finally becoming mainstream concerns, but it is very easy for us to expect that someone else – usually the 'they' embodied by local authorities, central government, scientists and people with more time on their hands – will sort this out. This is impossible. For one thing, habitat destruction is so casual and widespread that it is something all of us need to take seriously in our local areas. For another, the 'they' in positions of power can often make things worse. In 2012, Sheffield Council started felling trees in its streets, claiming that many of them were dying, diseased or dangerous, and that they needed replacing with saplings. Local campaigners argued that this was actually a cost-saving measure because the council didn't want to shell out on tree surgery or road modifications which would have meant the trees, some of which were old or rare, could have stayed. The campaigners eventually managed to halt the felling, but not before 5500 trees had been chainsawed down. The assumption which led to this programme was that streets were more important than trees, and that local people would value being able to park their car over the sight of a doughty elm which had survived Dutch elm disease.[6]

Perhaps the strength of feeling that the Sheffield tree-felling stirred up will serve as a warning to other local authorities tempted to think that the natural world is the least important part of the areas they serve. Politicians will change according to the mood of the electorate, and when plastic in the oceans becomes a talking point at water coolers, then it becomes a topic in national debate too. The more people who visit, value and celebrate their local green spaces, the more likely they are to stay safe. And given that the noisy people are often the ones who bother to complain about 'weeds' on grass verges or trees shading their cars, those of us who see these things as a vital part of our well-being need to shout even louder.

But our responsibility goes beyond making a noise. How many of us value our local green space but do little to keep it in good condition? Outdoor swimming groups sometimes organise litter picking sessions on the banks of and the waters in which they swim, having grown disgusted by the amount of rubbish discarded by others. In the summer, parks, beaches and nature reserves can become littered with the detritus of a good afternoon enjoyed by people who somehow feel entitled to leave their rubbish for someone else to pick up. This is clearly considered culturally acceptable by a large number of people, particularly given no one in a group thinks to object to their friends discarding drinks cans and food packages in the landscape they'd all turned up to enjoy.

We demand cheaper food, though we throw out a third of what we buy because we didn't need it anyway, and expect vegetables so perfect that supermarkets cancel orders on the basis of apples being 'too big', without regard for the impact that intensive agriculture has on the natural environment.[7] Rivers become polluted by run-off from fertilisers, rendering them not only dangerous for us to swim in, but also inhospitable to wildlife generally. Pesticides silence the hum of insects in the fields. This is not to denigrate farmers, by the way: they have merely responded to our mad demands for an unsustainable supply of food. Some are now trying to push back, 'rewilding' their farms as much as they can and focusing on quality of produce rather than quantity, but they can only go so far when consumers are still happy to switch their minds off when it comes to finding out how their food was produced.

We don't know what the countryside should look like any more. In her book *Wilding*, conservationist Isabella Tree describes the complaints she and her husband received when they decided to convert their farm at Knepp Castle into a 'rewilding' project.[8] Knepp is controversial in lots of ways, but a clearly specious complaint was that allowing scrub to grow and creeping thistles to flourish meant the landscape didn't 'look' like the countryside. Tree writes that the volume of angry letters slowly reduced as locals grew used to what nature really looked like, and saw the way painted ladies filled the air – and their larvae ate the thistles – or heard the calls of nightingales and turtle doves for the first time. But the visceral reaction to the removal of neat, bright green pasture and the messiness of real nature was telling: we don't even really know what 'natural' is any more.

We are very particular about the spaces that we own ourselves, but not always in a way that is conducive to a thriving Natural Health Service. How many of us coat our lawns in herbicides each year to remove the 'weeds', turning the garden into an ecological desert? What is the point of removing anything that isn't a grass, anyway? Of course, you don't want your lawn choked by bindweed, but there are many low-growing flowers which happily survive mowing and which turn your lawn from a boring carpet into a colourful tapestry: the purple-flowered self-heal, daisies, clover for the bees and buttercups. A living lawn moves and has a sound of its own, and yet we have become obsessed with controlling nature to the extent that we would rather our gardens were boring, just to prove that we are somehow the boss of all we see. There is also a growing enthusiasm for artificial grass lawns, which are, of course, weed-free and apparently perfect. So now, instead of mowing the lawn, gardeners vacuum clean it, and more and more scraps of plastic find their way into our natural world because of our desperate need for a smooth green sward. We spray our plants with pesticides rather than encourage a proper ecosystem in which predators will remove aphids and slugs, and tarmac over our front gardens so we have somewhere to park the car.

We have even become confused about what wildlife gardening is: many people think beekeeping is somehow a good thing for the environment when in fact honeybees are just one species of bee among around 270 in the UK, and they often outcompete other, threatened, bees when someone installs a new hive.

Changing to wildlife-friendly gardening isn't going to save the world, but the difference that it can make on even a small plot is impressive. If you stop being a control freak and encourage nature to help you garden you'll find that there are birds and hedgehogs keen to eat your slugs, that there are hoverflies and ladybirds chomping away at your aphids, and that you haven't killed off all the moths that might want to flutter around a honeysuckle in the evening. It means that even if you cannot leave the house, you can watch nature getting on with its day: I have written much of this book while watching goldfinches, blue tits, great tits, coal tits, sparrows, starlings, blackbirds and even a great spotted woodpecker enjoying the feeders I've installed in my small London back garden. Stacks of dead wood under bushes, leaving leaves to form a habitat and eventually rot down on the soil surface, and keeping a compost heap all make your garden more alive. Perhaps it is the life in the garden that many people fear, having grown so separated from nature that they don't want to share their lives with it at all.

Our separation from nature also makes us behave in utterly daft ways. I spend a lot of time walking my dog in Richmond Park, and enjoy sitting still to watch green woodpeckers, or yaffles, rootling about in the anthills for food, or listening to the tawny owl which I still haven't managed to spot hooting away high up in a tree. But I also find myself watching with horror as other people walk right up to the deer for selfies. I once went up to a couple approaching a large red stag, grinning and with a selfie stick ready, to explain to them that this magnificent beast weighed around 200 kilograms, could move at 40 miles per hour, and was so pumped full of testosterone that he would chase them and potentially even gore them. They were genuinely surprised: 'Oh, he looked so friendly,' said the woman, who was clearly so bewitched by his big brown eyes that she hadn't noticed his far bigger antlers. In the rutting season, when the stags are fighting over females, people end up being attacked in the Royal Parks, often because they have ignored the guidance to stay 100 metres away and not place themselves between a stag and a doe. It defies logic that someone wouldn't at least think twice about whether a creature as big and wild as a stag is safe to saunter up to, but it seems we have so removed ourselves from nature that we view it as a theme park existing for our social media channels, rather than something we might want to bother understanding.

Children

We aren't doing very much to stop the next generation from having
a similarly dysfunctional relationship with the natural world. Writer
Robert Macfarlane was troubled by the loss of natural words from
children's lexicons. The *Oxford Junior Dictionary* dropped the words
'acorn', 'bluebell' and 'kingfisher' because children didn't use them
enough, and replaced them with 'attachment', 'broadband' and
'voicemail'. In 2015, Macfarlane and an extraordinary list of writers
including Margaret Atwood, Michael Morpurgo and Sir Andrew
Motion wrote an open letter to Oxford University Press, arguing
that the words should stay in the dictionary. They expressed concern
that the words replacing natural vocabulary were 'associated with
the interior, solitary childhoods of today', and said:

> This is not a romantic desire to reflect the rosy memories of our own
> childhoods onto today's youngsters. There is a shocking, proven
> connection between the decline in natural play and the decline in
> children's wellbeing. Compared with a generation ago, when 40 per
> cent of children regularly played in natural areas, now only 10 per cent
> do so, while another 40 per cent never play anywhere outdoors. Ever.
> Obesity, anti-social behaviour, friendlessness and fear are the known
> consequences. The physical fitness of children is declining 9 per cent
> per decade, according to Public Health England.
>
> For the first time ever, children's life expectancy is lower than that
> of their parents – us. When, in 2007, the OJD made the changes,
> this connection was understood, but less well-publicised than now.

The research evidence showing the links between natural play and
wellbeing, and between disconnection from nature and social ills, is
mounting.[9]

It was a damning letter. Oxford University Press replied with a list
of the natural words that it had kept in the *OJD*, such as hibernate,
badger, dragonfly, robin and tadpole. The organisation also pointed
out, entirely reasonably, that 'all our dictionaries are designed to
reflect language as it is used, rather than seeking to prescribe certain
words or word usages'.[10] In other words, it wasn't the dictionary's
fault if no one was talking about kingfishers with their children.

Macfarlane then discovered a National Trust survey that found
half of children couldn't tell the difference between a wasp and a bee,
even though almost all of them could name a Dalek.[11] Troubled, too,
by the loss of habitats and species, he decided to write a book that
would encourage children to want to save nature. *The Lost Words* is
a book of spells and beautiful illustrations by artist Jackie Morris,
all aimed at teaching children just how magical a kingfisher really
is.[12] It has become so popular that there are now crowdfunding
campaigns around the country to get the book into every school,
with many of that fundraising citing children's mental health as a
key reason to reconnect pupils with nature.

As *The Lost Words* flies off the shelves, so big organisations and
public bodies are trying to reverse children's disconnect with nature.
The Wild Network was founded after a National Trust report
concluded that 'we as a nation, and especially our children, are
exhibiting symptoms of a modern phenomenon known as "Nature
Deficit Disorder"'.[13] It grew into a network of 30,000 people and

2000 organisations including the National Trust, RSPB, NHS and local government, and now tries to fight the barriers to getting children outdoors and in nature. Those barriers, according to work by the Wild Network, are fear, time, space and technology.[14] Fear includes the risk-averse culture and parents worrying that their children will encounter dangerous strangers, traffic or other hazards, including nature itself, if they are left to play in the great outdoors. Many parents don't have time to take their children outdoors, and there is precious little opportunity for unstructured outdoor play, either. The school curriculum is 'nature-starved', and not all individual schools are doing much to make up for that. Green spaces are vanishing and play is increasingly something that is commoditised: you have to buy a toy for a child to enjoy, rather than telling them to make their own fun in the outside world. And technology speaks for itself: children are spending more and more time parked in front of a screen.

The Wild Network produced a film called *Project Wild Thing*, which tried to persuade parents and children to get outdoors.[15] It also developed a free app called 'Wild Explorers', which shows parents how many outdoor activities there are – and how easy they are to do. Some of these take just ten minutes and are categorised as 'on our doorstep'. Others take several hours in a local woodland or park. The app is sponsored by Persil and bears the slogan 'Dirt is Good'.

The more time a child spends outdoors, the easier it is for a parent or guardian to introduce the idea of unstructured play. You don't need to give a child a set activity in a woodland, and nor do you need to fret about them tripping over logs or getting muddy. The

Forest School movement aims to connect children with nature as they learn, but it also places a great emphasis on letting children explore nature for themselves, rather than setting them a series of tasks. There are, though, many activities that families can do together outdoors. Local wildlife trusts run regular conservation days aimed at families. These are free and also improve a nature reserve or habitat by removing invasive species, stacking dead wood to create habitats for invertebrates and planting trees so that the shifting baseline is adjusted just a little. They also mean that nature becomes a part of growing up and of family life. It isn't something alien, distant or inaccessible. A study in 2016 by the Wild Network found that three-quarters of UK children spend less time outdoors than prison inmates, while analysis by Natural England in the same year discovered that more than one in nine children hadn't set foot in any sort of natural environment, including the humble local park, for at least twelve months.[16,17] The zone in which children are free to play, walk around and explore alone outside has shrunk dramatically with each generation. Words for birds, wild flowers and other natural terms have disappeared from children's dictionaries to reflect their growing irrelevance to most children's lives.

Given many naturalists say their love of the great outdoors was sparked in childhood, and given research suggests that the number of times a child visits a woodland has a direct correlation to the frequency of visits they make as an adult, this does not bode well for adults.[18] But it also does not bode well for the quality of life that children themselves have. If we accept that we need nature around us, then that doesn't just apply to adults, but to children, who are developing their sense of self, their coping strategies and their understanding of how to relax. Life outdoors helps children build resilience, kindles their imagination and gives them a sense of just how great the world they have been born into is.

It isn't clear whether we are experiencing what some have badged an 'explosion' of mental illness among young people, not least because more people may be both aware of what looks like poor mental health and also more prepared to talk about it. NHS England found a small rise in mental health problems in young people, from 11.4 per cent of under-sixteens in 1999 to 13.6 per cent in 2017.[19] That's not an 'explosion'. But it is also the case that there are a lot of children suffering from mental health problems who could well benefit from time outdoors. A report by the Children's Society in 2018 claimed that more than 100,000 children aged fourteen in the UK are self-harming, with 22 per cent of all girls of that age affected.[20] It may well be the case that there will always be a significant proportion of children who have a mental illness, regardless of the efforts we go to as a society. But can we really say we are giving children the best chance to be mentally healthy? I'm not sure that we are – and, of course, the less time we as adults spend in the great outdoors, the less likely our children are to see it as being an important part of life.

What About Indoors?

It's all very well going on about how much time someone spends outdoors. But all of us have to go inside at some point. We tend to see the built environment as being mutually exclusive with the great outdoors, concreting over meadows and shutting children in rooms rather than letting them roam in the woods. Cities, which are far more recent additions to the human experience than the natural world, are associated with higher rates of mental illness, with one meta-analysis finding that psychiatric disorders had a higher prevalence in urban areas than in rural areas.[21] There's even an illness caused by poorly-designed buildings. Sick building syndrome covers a range of symptoms people only experience when in a particular building, often their office. These include tiredness and difficulty concentrating; headaches; blocked nose; itchy skin or rashes; and dry eyes. But this is not inevitable: good town planning and architecture can enhance our enjoyment of the great outdoors, and mean that we spend more time experiencing it, whether under a roof or out in the open.

There is a think tank dedicated to studying how architecture and planning can improve – or damage – mental health. The Centre for Urban Design and Mental Health names aspects of the great outdoors as the first two things planners, designers and developers must consider. It has a framework called 'Mind the GAPS', with the G standing for 'green places' and A standing for 'active places' (P is for 'pro-social places' and S is 'safe places'). On the first, the Centre's policy brief says: 'access to natural settings in neighbourhoods and in the course of people's daily routines is likely to improve and maintain mental health and wellbeing'.[22]

Ben Channon is an architect who became interested in the impact buildings have on mental health when he was diagnosed with anxiety in his mid-twenties. He ended up writing a book, *Happy by Design*, which examines how to design with mental well-being in mind.[23] Unsurprisingly, natural light, greenery and easy access to exercise feature prominently. Channon worries that modern buildings often end up missing a number of these elements, with pressure not to include large windows, for instance, because of cost. This is particularly relevant in affordable housing, which has even higher budgetary pressures than other developments, and can be situated in less desirable areas.

Many years ago I used to be a housing journalist. One of the worst properties I ever visited was part of a prestigious central London development. A tenant in the social housing section – included as part of the conditions for granting planning permission – had contacted me in great distress because of the conditions he and his neighbours were being forced to live in. I was used to reporting on old, decrepit council flats with mould on the walls and thoughtlessly-designed dark corridors where antisocial behaviour flourishes, so I was rather baffled that these brand-new homes were apparently upsetting their residents so much. When I arrived, I discovered that the social block of flats was right at the back of the development, on the least desirable plot. This wasn't unusual, but, in this case, what made the land particularly unattractive was that it was right next to Victoria station, one of the busiest rail terminuses in the country. Trains were constantly screeching past all day and well into the night. The windows were tiny and looked out on to the railway. One windowpane had allegedly cracked as a result of the noise outside. Inside the flats, which had been designed to be as eco-efficient as possible, the tenants were boiling, to the extent that some claimed their children were suffering from regular nosebleeds. Many windows were overshadowed by other buildings or walls. It was particularly distressing for the tenant who I interviewed, because he had mental health problems relating to a serious trauma in his life. The regular awakenings during the night because of the trains reminded him of that trauma, and his health was deteriorating.

The tenants had little access to green space or even the outside. Their housing association had asked the architects not to include balconies when designing the block, because it feared they would use them for 'unsightly storage' (one of the elements of mindful design that Channon highlights is adequate storage, as a messy home is known to send the stress hormone cortisol surging). They couldn't access shared outdoor space made available to those living in the full-price properties. Bizarrely, despite the obvious misery of the tenants, this property actually won an award.

Given there are higher rates of mental illness among those on low incomes, this seems particularly unfair. It's also worth remembering that social housing was originally conceived by Octavia Hill, who believed passionately in the value of the great outdoors. She saw homes for the poor as a place where people could repair broken lives, not where the building itself could make someone sicker.

Planning goes beyond individual buildings and into the way our towns and cities are designed. It may well be the case that homes have a lot of green space nearby, but that it is very difficult for someone to get there safely on foot or by bike. If you don't have a car – or would rather cut down on emissions and do a bit more exercise – then you might not be able to get to that green space at all. British towns and cities lag miserably behind some of their European counterparts when it comes to cycling infrastructure, though London, Manchester and others have made significant improvements in recent years.

Most of us live in homes and on streets planned and built decades ago, so we cannot just focus on how new developments can improve mental health. There are ways of greening the existing built environment which don't cost a great deal and which have many of the additional benefits to mental health that we discovered in Chapter Two. Friends of the Earth runs a project called '10xGreener', which uses crowdfunding to pay for 'postcode gardeners'. These workers run community gardening projects which include making over front gardens and shared green spaces. The first postcode gardener was Kate Poland, appointed to the E5 postcode in London. She helped to change the way the local environment looked, hoping that by doing so, the mental and physical health of those living there would improve too.

And what about the places where people are treated for their mental health problems? We've visited the gardens and grounds of Bethlem, which are extraordinarily and famously beautiful. In some countries nature is considered such an important part of the healing process that hospitals are designed with it in mind. In Singapore, which has the highest number of mental health beds per population in the world, the Khoo Teck Puat Hospital building practises something called 'biophilic design integration', which is a fancy way of saying it incorporates greenery. The extent to which it does this is stunning: the total surface area of horizontal and vertical greenery is nearly four times the plot of land that the building occupies. Courtyards with plants including trees which rise through multiple levels of the hospital, balconies with scented plants, and water features all create a forest within this suburban site. It is also designed to give patients as much natural light as possible without sticking any of them in uncomfortable direct sunlight. There is a rooftop farm with fruit trees, vegetables and herbs, and other roof gardens for different wards.

Once again, many of our hospitals are housed in older buildings, and it is unrealistic to expect that they can be retrofitted with luxuriant greenery. But many hospitals do have charities supporting them which fundraise for better facilities for patients and their visiting relatives. Many of them are behind the beautiful gardens valued by patients, and the more emphasis these charitable groups are able to place on bringing nature into the hospital, the better.

And not just into the hospital, either. Maggie's Centres are charitable buildings always located near major cancer treatment hospitals. They offer emotional, practical and social support for people with cancer and their families, and are all designed with the natural environment as a key aspect of that support. Maggie's founder, Maggie Keswick Jencks, believed in the importance of 'a view out to trees, birds and sky' while people were being treated for cancer. The charity's architectural brief is exacting in its demands for these views, expecting landscape designers and architects to work together from the beginning, rather than seeing greenery as the boring evergreen stuff that gets bunged in at the end. It says:

> The interplay between outside and inside space, the built and the 'natural' environment is an important one. Sheltered inside, it helps to be reminded by a seasonal and changing scene outside, that you are still part of a living world…

> Sometimes, all that a person can bear, if they are in acute distress, is to look out of the window from a sheltered place, at the branch of a tree

moving in the wind. We would like there to be as many opportunities as possible to look out from wherever you are in the building, even if it is to an internal planted courtyard.[24]

Cancer can knock a person sideways mentally, with the effects lingering well into remission, and so the emphasis on natural views is not a luxury for Maggie's Centres; it is a core part of their support, as they work alongside hospitals.

Who Benefits?

Nature is free and all around us. That is a fact, but it is also true that the Natural Health Service runs the same risk of becoming something middle-class people use to treat their mental illnesses. Disadvantaged and minority groups are already less likely to access the great outdoors. A study run by government agency Natural England in 2015 of around 45,000 people found that minority ethnic groups, people living in deprived urban areas, disadvantaged social groups, over-sixty-fives and disabled people were all less likely to visit green spaces.[25] Reasons for not doing so included fears about safety, inadequate facilities and poor maintenance. These kinds of things matter if, for instance, you use a wheelchair and the paths are full of craters, there is no way of getting past the steps into the bird hide, or you cannot use a toilet. Disabled birdwatchers also complain that there is too much of a focus on wheelchair accessibility at the expense of other needs: few reserves have places for people to sit and rest if they have to walk a long stretch to the next bird hide, and signs are very rarely composed with the needs of people with sensory problems in mind. Similarly, elderly people often choose not to leave their homes if they do not think they will be able to visit a toilet while they are out.

It's also harder to access green space if you are poor: a 2014 study found that the most affluent 20 per cent of wards in England had five times the amount of green space than the most deprived 10 per cent of wards.[26] This is not just a matter for town planners, but also those working in existing communities, including GPs and local authorities. Is there sufficient access to allotments? Is there derelict land which can be converted – even for a short period of time – to a community garden? Are the people who live in that deprived area aware of the green space they have, and are they being encouraged to use it? Why is it that so many local authority and housing association estates display signs saying 'NO BALL GAMES'? Do those estates have any outdoor gyms, or even areas where you can play a ball game? Why are so many estates planted with shrubs that are spiky and uninviting, suggesting that nature is something best avoided as it might hurt you?

There's nothing wrong, of course, with the middle classes turning to the great outdoors. It's just that this NHS is supposed to be universally accessible like its namesake. And it is generally the case that we don't need to worry about whether the middle classes will find out about or be able to afford something that will help them. Getting other groups to use the Natural Health Service takes more effort.

Parkrun is one example of a natural health service which initially had a very middle-class appeal that is trying to reach out into deprived communities. Because of the way it grew, it tended to attract those already comfortable with the idea of going for a run and able to afford kit which made going for a run comfortable. And new parkruns tended to spring up in middle-class areas. But as it went from a raggle-taggle of volunteers to an organisation with full-time staff, it started to change the way it expanded. Parkrun deliberately tried to move into deprived communities. Some parkruns even organised clothing collections so that would-be runners had something to wear that made them fit in. Similarly, Operation Centaur was set up not as a stable that would engage people who already knew and loved horses, but to reach out to those who would benefit from their first ever contact with gentle giants. Such broad inclusion should serve as an example to others.

Beyond the voluntary sector, local authorities have an important role to play in ensuring that every section of society really benefits from the Natural Health Service. Some already do that very well. In fact, in the north-west of England, there is already something called the Natural Health Service, which offers many of the activities detailed in this book. It is part of the Mersey Forest, which was set up as a partnership of councils across Merseyside and North Cheshire over twenty-five years ago. The Natural Health Service focuses its efforts on areas of high health deprivation to reduce inequalities and works with veterans, carers, socially isolated people, obese adults, care leavers and unemployed men. It aims to keep people well, rather than to offer specific mental health treatment, and it tends not to promote its activities as being specifically for mental well-being, as this may put off the very people it is trying to target. Clare Olver, Natural Health Service Manager at the Mersey

Forest, says: 'It's about using the natural environment to improve the health and well-being of individuals.'

This approach to names is important. There are certain groups who love attending groups explicitly for their mental health which use all sorts of jargon about mindfulness and therapy, but there are many people who would run a mile from this or find it totally inaccessible. I did find some of the activities I joined while researching this book had a very middle-class feel merely because of the use of this jargon around 'invitations', the 'present moment' and so on. Again, there is nothing wrong with that if it helps a certain group. But it must be the case that our Natural Health Service is available and attractive to all, regardless of their background.

A New Perspective

My day visiting the lady's-slipper orchid in 2017 might have seemed like a luxury to many onlookers. How could I be that unwell if I was driving myself to a nature reserve and photographing a silly plant? Even the story of said silly plant seems a bit over the top: it is thanks to a £1 million endowment that scientists at Kew were able to work out how to get its seeds to germinate. A great deal of money is spent on the fortress protecting the one surviving plant in the Yorkshire Dales, on the reintroduction of the orchid to other sites and on maintaining those sites. What a lot of effort, just to protect one little bit of nature.

And the effort to protect the Natural Health Service might seem similarly over the top. Aren't there more urgent things to be spending money and time on? Yes, trees are nice and gardens are good, but what about our education, our hospitals, our workplaces?

It isn't the case, though, that we can separate those things, or at least it shouldn't be. We have tried very hard to fence ourselves away from the great outdoors, seeing it as something either to be feared or only used if you earn a certain amount of money and live somewhere a bit posh. We have made it out to be as silly and luxurious an optional extra as the lady's-slipper orchid, which is a wonderful rarity but, like so many very rare plants, hardly plays an integral role in an ecosystem. But in adopting this attitude, we have tried to cut our umbilical cord with the natural world and things aren't working out for us as a result.

We have met so many people, whether expert in a field or expert in their own personal illness, who have seen the way the outdoors can help their minds. No, they haven't been transformed into totally healthy people. Yes, illnesses are crafty and can circumvent the good work of the Natural Health Service, just as physical illnesses can make a mockery of the most advanced drugs on offer. But time and again an intervention from the great outdoors has made treatment that bit easier, life worth living and symptoms that bit less all-consuming. And the exciting thing is that we do not know even the half of it yet. We are just starting to see small glimmers of light, like the sun filtering through to the woodland floor, of what we might be able to achieve using our innate need for nature.

And if we really do need nature to live well, whether that be with a mental health problem or with a luckily healthy mind, then we need to behave as though that really is the case. It simply isn't an optional extra. It isn't something to fit into our lives, but something that we should be fitting our lives around, whether that be through the way doctors treat their mentally ill patients, how we design the buildings and towns we live in, or the effort we put into protecting the natural environment. We have to see the Natural Health Service as something integral to our way of life. Instead of looking for ways to let nature in, we should be asking why our default when designing anything, whether it be a physical building or a theoretical system, is to shut nature out.

The consequences of a fully-functioning Natural Health Service could be magnificent. In some cases, people wouldn't need the acute interventions and medication that doctors find themselves with no choice but to offer. It would be prevention for many and cure for others. This would save money, far more than the sums spent protecting rare plants from loose-fingered humans. But it would do more than that. Money is a good thing to save, for sure. But there's nothing more astounding than the prospect of saving a life. Even the glory of nature comes second to that.

References

CHAPTER ONE: Why We Need Nature

1 Plato. *The Republic*, book 3, section 411e.
2 Walker, D., 2018. *Walker's Manly Exercises*. Penguin Books [Kindle edition], p. 12.
3 Hill, O., 1883. *Homes of the London Poor*.
4 Ulrich, R. S., 1984. View through a window may influence recovery from surgery. *Science*, 27;224(4647), pp. 420–1.
5 Moore, E. O., 1981. A prison environment's effect on health care service demands. *Journal of Environmental Systems*, 11(1), pp. 17–34.
6 Hunter, M. R., Gillespie, B. W. and Chen, S. Y. P., 2019. Urban nature experiences reduce stress in the context of daily life based on salivary biomarkers. *Frontiers in Psychology*, 10, p. 722.
7 Joye, Y. and Bolderdijk, J. W., 2015. An exploratory study into the effects of extraordinary nature on emotions, mood, and prosociality. *Frontiers in Psychology*, 5, p. 1577.
8 Barton, J. and Pretty, J., 2010. What is the best dose of nature and green exercise for improving mental health? A multi-study analysis. *Environmental Science and Technology*, 44(10), pp. 3947–55.
9 Kellert, S. R. and Wilson, E. O. (eds.), 1995. *The Biophilia Hypothesis*. Island Press, p. 32 [Kindle edition].
10 Kaplan, R. and Kaplan, S., 1989. *The Experience of Nature: A Psychological Perspective*. Cambridge University Press.
11 Mayer, F. S., Frantz, C. M., Bruehlman-Senecal, E. and Dolliver, K., 2009. Why is nature beneficial? The role of connectedness to nature. *Environment and Behavior*, 41(5), pp. 607–43.

12 Bromley by Bow Centre. Social prescribing April 2017–March 2018. Retrieved from https://www.bbbc.org.uk/wp-content/uploads/2018/08/Tower-Hamlets-Social-Prescribing-Report-Apr-Mar-2018-.pdf.

13 Parkinson, H. J., 30 Jun. 2018. 'It's nothing like a broken leg': Why I'm done with the mental health conversation. *Guardian*.

CHAPTER TWO: Sowing the Seeds of Sanity

1 Hickman, C., 2014. Cheerfulness and tranquility: Gardens in the Victorian asylum. *The Lancet Psychiatry*, *1*(7), pp. 506–7.

2 Don, M., March 2019. *BBC Gardeners' World Magazine*.

3 Lowry, C. A., Hollis, J. H., De Vries, A., Pan, B., Brunet, L. R., Hunt, J. R., Paton, J. F., van Kampen, E., Knight, D. M., Evans, A. K. and Rook, G. A., 2007. Identification of an immune-responsive mesolimbocortical serotonergic system: potential role in regulation of emotional behavior. *Neuroscience*, *146*(2), pp. 756–72.

4 Clatworthy, J., Hinds, J. and M. Camic, P., 2013. Gardening as a mental health intervention: A review. *Mental Health Review Journal*, *18*(4), pp. 214–25.

5 Buck, D., May 2016. Gardens and health: Implications for policy and practice. The King's Fund. Retrieved from https://www.kingsfund.org.uk/sites/default/files/field/field_publication_file/Gardens_and_health.pdf.

6 Schillinger, N., 2013. *Veg Street*. Short Books, p. 8.

7 Bringslimark, T., Hartig, T. and Patil, G. G., 2009. The psychological benefits of indoor plants: A critical review of the experimental literature. *Journal of Environmental Psychology*, *29*(4), pp. 422–33.

8 Lee, M. S., Lee, J., Park, B. J. and Miyazaki, Y., 2015. Interaction with indoor plants may reduce psychological and physiological stress by suppressing autonomic nervous system activity in young adults: A randomized crossover study. *Journal of Physiological Anthropology*, *34*(1), p. 21.

CHAPTER THREE: Obsessing About Nature

1 Kabat-Zinn, J., 2005. *Wherever You Go, There You Are: Mindfulness Meditation in Everyday Life*. Hachette Books.

2 Williams, J. M. G., Crane, C., Barnhofer, T., Brennan, K., Duggan, D. S., Fennell, M. J., Hackmann, A., Krusche, A., Muse, K., Von Rohr, I. R. and

Shah, D., 2014. Mindfulness-based cognitive therapy for preventing relapse in recurrent depression: A randomized dismantling trial. *Journal of Consulting and Clinical Psychology*, *82*(2), p. 275.

3   Querstret, D., Cropley, M. and Fife-Schaw, C., 2018. The effects of an online mindfulness intervention on perceived stress, depression and anxiety in a non-clinical sample: A randomised waitlist control trial. *Mindfulness*, *9*(6), pp. 1825–36.

4   Mental Health Foundation, 2010. Mindfulness Report 2010. Retrieved from https://www.mentalhealth.org.uk/sites/default/files/Mindfulness_report_2010.pdf.

5   Mindfulness All-Party Parliamentary Group, Oct. 2015. Mindful Nation UK. Retrieved from https://www.themindfulnessinitiative.org/Handlers/Download.ashx?IDMF=1af56392-4cf1-4550-bdd1-72e809fa627a.

6   Mabey, R., 2011. *Nature Cure*. Vintage Digital [Kindle edition].

7   Mental Health Foundation, 2011. Learning for life: Adult learning, mental health and wellbeing. Retrieved from https://www.mentalhealth.org.uk/sites/default/files/learning-for-life.pdf.

8   Oswald, A., 2010. *Dart*. Faber & Faber [Kindle edition].

9   McCullough, M. E. and Emmons, R. A., 2003. Counting blessings versus burdens: An experimental investigation of gratitude and subjective well-being in daily life. *Journal of Personality and Social Psychology*, *84*(2), pp. 377–89.

10 Zahn, R., Moll, J., Paiva, M., Garrido, G., Krueger, F., Huey, E. D. and Grafman, J., 2008. The neural basis of human social values: Evidence from functional MRI. *Cerebral Cortex*, *19*(2), pp. 276–83.

11 Cotman, C. W. and Berchtold, N. C., 2002. Exercise: A behavioral intervention to enhance brain health and plasticity. *Trends in Neurosciences*, *25*(6), pp. 295–301.

12 Gourgouvelis, J., Yielder, P. and Murphy, B., 2017. Exercise promotes neuroplasticity in both healthy and depressed brains: An fMRI pilot study. *Neural Plasticity*, *2017*, 8305287.

CHAPTER FOUR: Walking the Black Dog

1   Wainwright, A., 2005. *A Pictorial Guide to the Lakeland Fells: Book 7*. Frances Lincoln.

2   Keats, J., 2003. *The Complete Poems*. Penguin Books [Kindle edition].

3   Li, Q., 2019. *Shinrin-Yoku: The Healing Art of Forest Bathing*.

Penguin Books [Kindle edition], p. 95.

4 Kotte, D., Li, Q. and Shin, W. S. (eds.), 2019. *International Handbook of Forest Therapy*. Cambridge Scholars Publishing, p. 132.

5 Komori, T., Fujiwara, R., Tanida, M., Nomura, J. and Yokoyama, M. M., 1995. Effects of citrus fragrance on immune function and depressive states. *Neuroimmunomodulation*, 2(3), pp. 174–80.

6 Li, Q., 2019. *Shinrin-Yoku: The Healing Art of Forest Bathing*. Penguin Books [Kindle edition], p. 118.

7 Williams, F., 2017. *The Nature Fix: Why Nature Makes Us Happier, Healthier, and More Creative*. W. W. Norton & Company [Kindle edition], p. 144.

8 Wilson, N., Jun. 2009. Branching out: Greenspace and conservation on referral. Forestry Commission Scotland. Retrieved from https://forestry.gov.scot/publications/320-branching-out-evaluation-2009-full-report/viewdocument; CJC Consulting, May 2016. Branching out economic study extension: Final report. Forestry Commission Scotland. Retrieved from https://forestry.gov.scot/images/corporate/pdf/branching-out-report-2016.pdf.

9 Coillte. Woodlands for health: Summary report. Retrieved from http://www.wicklowmentalhealth.org/images/pdf/Projects-Woodlands-For-Health-Summary-Report.pdf.

10 The Marmot Review, Feb. 2010. Fair society, healthy lives. Institute of Health Equity. Retrieved from http://www.instituteofhealthequity.org/resources-reports/fair-society-healthy-lives-the-marmot-review/fair-society-healthy-lives-full-report-pdf.pdf.

11 Li, Q., 2019. *Shinrin-Yoku: The Healing Art of Forest Bathing*. Penguin Books [Kindle edition], p. 121.

12 Wohlleben, P., 2017. *The Hidden Life of Trees: What They Feel, How They Communicate: Discoveries from a Secret World*. William Collins [Kindle edition].

13 Ofcom, 2 Aug. 2018. Communications Market Report. Retrieved from https://www.ofcom.org.uk/__data/assets/pdf_file/0022/117256/CMR-2018-narrative-report.pdf.

14 Richardson, M., Hussain, Z. and Griffiths, M. D. (2018). Problematic smartphone use, nature connectedness, and anxiety. *Journal of Behavioral Addictions*, 7(1), pp. 109–16.

15 Hymas, C., 2 Aug. 2018. Government should tell parents not to give smartphones to under-11s, says leading psychiatrist. *Telegraph*.

16 Pitchforth, J., Fahy, K., Ford, T., Wolpert, M., Viner, R. M.

and Hargreaves, D.S., 2019. Mental health and well-being trends among children and young people in the UK, 1995–2014: Analysis of repeated cross-sectional national health surveys. *Psychological Medicine, 49*(8), pp. 1275–85.

17 Radiological Society of North America, 30 Nov. 2017. Smartphone addiction creates imbalance in brain. Retrieved from https://press.rsna.org/timssnet/media/pressreleases/14_pr_target.cfm?ID=1989.

18 Christensen, M. A., Bettencourt, L., Kaye, L., Moturu, S. T., Nguyen, K. T., Olgin, J. E., Pletcher, M. J. and Marcus, G. M., 2016. Direct measurements of smartphone screen-time: Relationships with demographics and sleep. *PloS One, 11*(11), p. e0165331

CHAPTER FIVE: Racing Out of the Darkness

1 Virgo, H., 2017. *Stand Tall Little Girl: Facing Up to Anorexia.* Trigger Publishing.

2 Mackie, B., 2018. *Jog On: How Running Saved My Life.* HarperCollins Publishers [Kindle edition], pp. 12–13.

3 Gordon, B., 2018. *Eat, Drink, Run: How I Got Fit Without Going Too Mad.* Headline [Kindle edition].

4 Hewitt, P., 2019. *Outrunning the Demons: Lives Transformed Through Running.* Bloomsbury Sport.

5 Murakami, H., 2011. *What I Talk About When I Talk About Running.* Random House [Kindle edition], p. 17.

6 Agudelo, L. Z., Femenía, T., Orhan, F., Porsmyr-Palmertz, M., Goiny, M., Martinez-Redondo, V., Correia, J. C., Izadi, M., Bhat, M., Schuppe-Koistinen, I. and Pettersson, A. T., 2014. Skeletal muscle PGC-1α1 modulates kynurenine metabolism and mediates resilience to stress-induced depression. *Cell, 159*(1), pp. 33–45.

7 Hanson, N. J., Short, L. E., Flood, L. T., Cherup, N. P. and Miller, M. G., 2018. Cortical neural arousal is differentially affected by type of physical exercise performed. *Experimental Brain Research, 236*(6), pp. 1643–9.

8 Firth, J., Stubbs, B., Vancampfort, D., Schuch, F., Lagopoulos, J., Rosenbaum, S. and Ward, P. B., 2018. Effect of aerobic exercise on hippocampal volume in humans: A systematic review and meta-analysis. *Neuroimage, 166*, pp. 230–8.

9 Morris, P., 2017. Not just a run in the park: A qualitative exploration of parkrun and mental health. Staffordshire University & Keele University [doctoral thesis]

CHAPTER SIX: Cold Water That Warms the Soul

1 Heminsley, A., 2017. *Leap In: A Woman, Some Waves, and the Will to Swim*. Random House [Kindle edition].

2 Deakin, R., 2000. *Waterlog: A Swimmer's Journey Through Britain*. Vintage.

3 Nichols, G., 1984. *The Fat Black Woman's Poems*. Virago Poets.

4 Pantzar, K., 2018. *Finding Sisu: In Search of Courage, Strength and Happiness the Finnish Way*. Hodder & Stoughton [Kindle edition].

5 Massey, H. and Scully, P. [no date]. How to acclimatise to cold water. The Outdoor Swimming Society. Retrieved from https://www.outdoorswimmingsociety.com/how-to-acclimatise-to-cold-water/.

6 Janský, L., Pospíšilová, D., Honzova, S., Uličný, B., Šrámek, P., Zeman, V. and Kaminkova, J., 1996. Immune system of cold-exposed and cold-adapted humans. *European Journal of Applied Physiology and Occupational Physiology*, 72(5–6), pp. 445–50.

7 Buckley, J. P. D., 2015. *Cool Swimming: A Quick Dip Into Cold Water Swimming and Physical and Mental Well-Being*. CreateSpace.

8 Radboud University Nijmegen Medical Centre, 2011. Research on 'Iceman' Wim Hof suggests it may be possible to influence autonomic nervous system and immune response. ScienceDaily. Retrieved from https://www.sciencedaily.com/releases/2011/04/110422090203.htm.

9 Bullmore, E., 2019. *The Inflamed Mind: A Radical New Approach to Depression*. Short Books Ltd.

10 Golden, F. S. and Tipton, M. J., 1988. Human adaptation to repeated cold immersions. *The Journal of Physiology*, 396(1), pp. 349–63.

11 Siems, W. G., van Kuijk, F. J., Maass, R. and Brenke, R., 1994. Uric acid and glutathione levels during short-term whole body cold exposure. *Free Radical Biology and Medicine*, 16(3), pp. 299–305.

12 Schniepp, J., Campbell, T. S., Powell, K. L. and Pincivero, D. M., 2002. The effects of cold-water immersion on power output and heart rate in elite cyclists. *Journal of Strength and Conditioning Research*, 16(4), pp. 561–6.

13 Šrámek, P., Šimečková, M., Janský, L., Šavlíková, J. and Vybíral, S., 2000. Human physiological responses to immersion into water of different temperatures. *European Journal of Applied Physiology*, 81(5), pp. 436–42.

14 *The Doctor Who Gave Up Drugs*. BBC One, 15 Sep. 2016.

CHAPTER SEVEN: All Creatures Great and Sane

1 Willingham, E., 28 Mar. 2019. Dogs detect the scent of seizures. *Scientific American.* Retrieved from https://www.scientificamerican.com/article/dogs-detect-the-scent-of-seizures/.

2 Beetz, A., 27 Nov. 2013. Socio-emotional correlates of a schooldog-teacher-team in the classroom. *Frontiers in Psychology.* Retrieved from https://www.frontiersin.org/articles/10.3389/fpsyg.2013.00886/full.

3 Kamioka, H., Okada, S., Tsutani, K., Park, H., Okuizumi, H., Handa, S., Oshio, T., Park, S. J., Kitayuguchi, J., Abe, T. and Honda, T., 2014. Effectiveness of animal-assisted therapy: A systematic review of randomized controlled trials. *Complementary Therapies in Medicine*, *22*(2), pp. 371–90.

4 Nimer, J. and Lundahl, B., 2007. Animal-assisted therapy: A meta-analysis. *Anthrozoös*, *20*(3), pp. 225–38.

5 Lloyd, J., Johnston, L. and Lewis, J., 6 Jun. 2019. Psychiatric assistance dog use for people living with mental health disorders. *Frontiers in Veterinary Science.* Retrieved from https://www.frontiersin.org/articles/10.3389/fvets.2019.00166/full.

6 Durcan, G., Dec. 2018. Restoring something lost: The mental health impact of therapy dogs in prisons. Centre for Mental Health. Retrieved from https://www.centreformentalhealth.org.uk/sites/default/files/2018-12/CentreforMentalHealth_Restoring_something_lost.pdf.

7 Durcan, G., Dec. 2018. Restoring something lost. Centre for Mental Health. Retrieved from https://www.centreformentalhealth.org.uk/sites/default/files/2018-12/CentreforMentalHealth_Restoring_something_lost.pdf.

8 Cats Protection League, 12 Jan. 2012. Purring the blues away. Retrieved from https://www.cats.org.uk/mediacentre/pressreleases/purring-the-blues-away.

9 Cited on Eagala's home page: https://www.eagala.org/.

10 Cantin, A. and Marshall-Lucette, S., 2011. Examining the literature on the efficacy of Equine Assisted Therapy for people with mental health and behavioural disorders. *Mental Health and Learning Disabilities Research and Practice*, *8*(1), pp. 51–61.

11 Canadian Agency for Drugs and Technologies in Health, 10 Aug. 2012. Therapy dogs and horses for mental health: A review of the clinical effectiveness. Retrieved from https://www.cadth.ca/media/pdf/htis/aug-2012/RC0381%20Therapy%20Animals%20final.pdf.

12 Nurenberg, J. R., Schleifer, S. J., Shaffer, T. M., Yellin, M., Desai,

P. J., Amin, R., Bouchard, A. and Montalvo, C., 2014. Animal-assisted therapy with chronic psychiatric inpatients: Equine-assisted psychotherapy and aggressive behavior. *Psychiatric Services, 66*(1), pp. 80–6.

13 Coffin, J., 2019. The Nguudu Barndimanmanha Project – improving social and emotional wellbeing in aboriginal youth through equine assisted learning. *Frontiers in Public Health, 7.*

14 Wells, T., Doran, S.-P. and Mayer, C., 6 Apr. 2016. The shireshank redemption: Storm as women lags get horses for 'therapy'. *Sun.*

15 Riding for the Disabled Association, 2018. Making a difference: Our impact 2018. Retrieved from https://www.rda.org.uk/wp-content/uploads/2019/05/RDA-Impact-2018.pdf.

16 Gawande, A., 2014. *Being Mortal: Illness, Medicine and What Matters In the End.* Wellcome Collection [Kindle edition], p.122.

17 Cook, G., Cook, M., Thynne, E. and Chandler, C., Sep. 2013. An evaluation of 'HENPOWER': Improving wellbeing & social capital in care settings. Equal Arts. Retrieved from https://equalarts.org.uk/media/HENPOWERfinalreport.pdf.

18 Holt-Lunstad, J., Smith, T. B. and Layton, J. B., 2010. Social relationships and mortality risk: A meta-analytic review. *PLoS Medicine, 7*(7), p. e1000316.

19 Nagesh, A., 12 Oct. 2018. Woman's emotional support squirrel kicked off flight. BBC Three. Retrieved from https://www.bbc.co.uk/bbcthree/article/39a2a5b9-9eea-4666-b5b5-fa3223ae248a.

20 BBC News, 31 Jan. 2018. 'Emotional support peacock' barred from United Airlines plane. Retrieved from https://www.bbc.co.uk/news/world-us-canada-42880690.

CHAPTER EIGHT: Does It Really Work?

1 Goldacre, B., 2008. *Bad Science.* HarperCollins [Kindle edition].

2 Fournier, J. C., DeRubeis, R. J., Hollon, S. D., Dimidjian, S., Amsterdam, J. D., Shelton, R. C. and Fawcett, J., 2010. Antidepressant drug effects and depression severity: A patient-level meta-analysis. *JAMA, 303*(1), pp. 47–53.

3 Evans, D., 2014. *Placebo: Mind Over Matter in Modern Medicine.* HarperCollins [Kindle edition].

4 MQ: Transforming Mental Health [no date]. How much is spent on mental health research in the UK? Retrieved from https://www.mqmentalhealth.org/research/research-funding-landscape.

5 The Mental Health Taskforce, Feb. 2016. The five year forward view for mental health. Retrieved from https://www.england.nhs.uk/wp-content/uploads/2016/02/Mental-Health-Taskforce-FYFV-final.pdf.

6 Personal Social Services Research Unit [no date]. NHS reference costs for mental health services. Retrieved from https://www.pssru.ac.uk/wp-content/uploads/2017/10/2.1-NHS-reference-costs-for-mental-health-services.pdf.

7 Mental Health America, 2019. The state of mental health in America: 2019. Retrieved from https://mhanational.org/sites/default/files/2019%20MH%20in%20America%20Final_0.pdf.

8 Mitchell, E., 2018. *The Wild Remedy: How Nature Mends Us – A Diary*. Michael O'Mara [Kindle edition], p. xxxvi.

9 Strayed, C., 2012. *Wild: A Journey from Lost to Found*. Atlantic Books.

10 Deakin, R., 2011. *Waterlog: A Swimmer's Journey Through Britain*. Random House [Kindle edition].

11 Minihane, J., 2017. *Floating: A Return to Waterlog*. Duckworth [Kindle edition].

CHAPTER NINE: The Natural Health Service: A Manifesto

1 NHS, 2 Mar. 2018. Homeopathy. Retrieved from https://www.nhs.uk/conditions/homeopathy/; NHS England [no date]. Items which should not be routinely prescribed in primary care. Retrieved from https://www.england.nhs.uk/medicines/items-which-should-not-be-routinely-prescribed/.

2 Stevenson, D. and Farmer, P., Oct. 2017. Thriving at work: The Stevenson/Farmer review of mental health and employers. Retrieved from https://assets.publishing.service.gov.uk/government/uploads/system/uploads/attachment_data/file/658145/thriving-at-work-stevenson-farmer-review.pdf.

3 Ibid.

4 McCarthy, M., 2015. *The Moth Snowstorm: Nature and Joy*. John Murray.

5 Ibid.

6 Drury, C., 12 Apr. 2018. Sheffield's tree massacre: How locals battled to protect Europe's greenest city. *Independent*. Retrieved from https://www.independent.co.uk/news/long_reads/sheffield-tree-massacre-parks-green-city-spaces-felling-street-council-yorkshire-a8286581.html.

7 Fogle, B., 28 Nov. 2019. These apples have been left to rot… [tweet]. Twitter. Retrieved from https://twitter.com/benfogle/status/1199980207614152705.

8 Tree, I., 2018. *Wilding: The Return of Nature to a British Farm.* Picador.

9 Furness, H., 12 Jan. 2015. Atwood, Morpurgo and Motion join campaign to bring nature back to children's dictionary. *Telegraph.* Retrieved from https://www.telegraph.co.uk/news/celebritynews/11341311/Atwood-Morpurgo-and-Motion-join-campaign-to-bring-nature-back-to-childrens-dictionary.html.

10 Flood, A., 13 Jan. 2015. Oxford Junior Dictionary's replacement of 'natural' words with 21st-century terms sparks outcry. *Guardian.* Retrieved from https://www.theguardian.com/books/2015/jan/13/oxford-junior-dictionary-replacement-natural-words.

11 Moss, S., 2012. Natural childhood. National Trust. Retrieved from https://nt.global.ssl.fastly.net/documents/read-our-natural-childhood-report.pdf.

12 Morris, J. and Macfarlane, R., 2017. *The Lost Words.* Hamish Hamilton.

13 Moss, S., 2012. Natural childhood. National Trust. Retrieved from https://nt.global.ssl.fastly.net/documents/read-our-natural-childhood-report.pdf.

14 The Wild Network [no date]. #WildTime. Retrieved from https://www.thewildnetwork.com/about.

15 The Wild Network [no date]. Project wild thing [video]. Retrieved from https://www.

thewildnetwork.com/inspiration/project-wild-thing.

16 Persil [no date]. Free the kids. Retrieved from https://www.persil.com/uk/free-the-kids.html.

17 Natural England, 10 Feb. 2016. Monitor of engagement with the natural environment pilot study: Visits to the natural environment by children. Gov. uk. Retrieved from https://www.gov.uk/government/statistics/monitor-of-engagement-with-the-natural-environment-pilot-study-visits-to-the-natural-environment-by-children.

18 Thompson, C. W., Aspinall, P. and Montarzino, A., 2008. The childhood factor: Adult visits to green places and the significance of childhood experience. *Environment and Behavior, 40*(1), pp. 111–43.

19 NHS Digital, 22 Nov. 2018. Mental health of children and young people in England, 2017. Retrieved from https://digital.nhs.uk/data-and-information/publications/statistical/mental-health-of-children-and-young-people-in-england/2017/2017.

20 The Children's Society, 2018. The good childhood report 2018. Retrieved from https://www.childrenssociety.org.uk/sites/default/files/the_good_childhood_report_full_2018.pdf.

21 Peen, J., Schoevers, R. A., Beekman, A. T. and Dekker, J., 2010. The current status of urban–rural differences in

psychiatric disorders. *Acta Psychiatrica Scandinavica, 121*(2), pp. 84–93.

22 The Centre for Urban Design and Mental Health [no date]. How urban design can impact mental health. Retrieved from https://www.urbandesignmentalhealth.com/how-urban-design-can-impact-mental-health.html.

23 Channon, B., 2018. *Happy by Design: A Guide to Architecture and Mental Wellbeing.* RIBA Publishing.

24 Maggie's Centres [no date]. Maggie's architecture and landscape brief. Retrieved from https://www.maggiescentres.org/media/uploads/publications/other-publications/Maggies_architecturalbrief_2015.pdf.

25 Natural England, 14 Jan. 2015. Monitor engagement with the natural environment: Annual report from the 2013–2014 survey (JP009). Retrieved from http://publications.natural england.org.uk/publication/6579788732956672?category=47018.

26 Public Health England, 8 Sep. 2014. Local action on health inequalities: Improving access to green spaces. Retrieved from https://assets.publishing.service.gov.uk/government/uploads/system/uploads/attachment_data/file/357411/Review8_Green_spaces_health_inequalities.pdf.

Acknowledgements

So many people made this book possible:

Those who were kind and bold enough to let me interview them about their mental illnesses.

The people who treat them and see the great outdoors as something to get excited about, even when working with the darkest conditions.

My agent Andrew Gordon for once again taking a scatty idea of mine and working out how it could become a book with a chance of being read.

Mike Harpley at Atlantic for being an even better editor this second time around than on the first book, for humouring my enthusiasm for bizarre pursuits in this book, and for very gently suggesting that maybe seventy-three mentions of orchids might be a tad excessive.

My editor at the *Spectator*, Fraser Nelson, has been a wonderful boss and mentor to me over many years now, and not only helped me stay in work when I was desperately ill but has also, I hope, provided a blueprint for other employers whose staff develop mental illnesses. I will always be so grateful for his support.

I couldn't have written this book, or frankly stayed alive, without my partner John Woodcock. Woodcocks are rare birds and worthy of celebration whenever they are found. John is the rarest of all, most importantly in his desire to help me savour my liberty and the pursuit of happiness after the darkest of times. And for putting up with four-hour walks to find orchids.

My parents, my brothers and my closest friends have all endured a great deal, not just as a result of me being unwell, but also because they have had to relive some of the hardest moments in this book.

I hope that, at the very least, what I have written will help other deeply worried families and friends know how they might help their loved ones when they find themselves in the black hole. It never lasts as long as your illness tells you it will.

Index